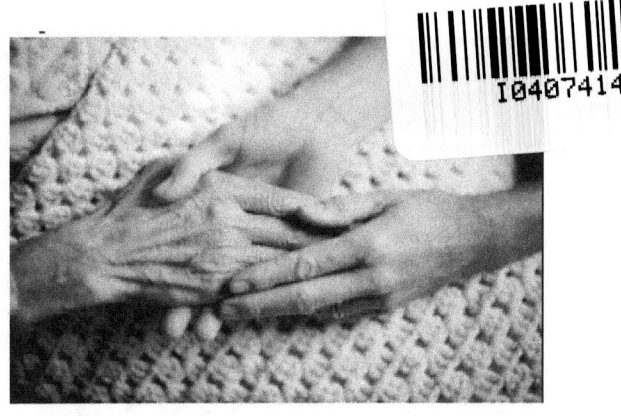

Coping with Caregiving

A Beginner's Guide to Becoming a Caregiver for Your Loved Ones Without Suffering from Caregiver Burnout

Annabelle Stevens

Carolyn Stone

Eternal Spiral Books

ISBN-13: 978-1540794956

ISBN-10: 1540794954

Eternal Spiral Books
NY, NY
http://EternalSpiralBooks.com/
Please visit us for a free newsletter, special offers and more.

DEDICATION

To Gran, disabled for over 40 years after a car accident, who never stopped laughing and living life to the full.

To Gramps, who cared for her so well until the day she died, but neglected to go to the doctor himself until it was too late.

To Grandpa, who had so many gallbladder surgeries he joked they should just give him a zipper in his abdomen.

To my father-in-law Bill, a hypochondriac who turned out to be the bravest man I ever met when it came to his liver cancer diagnosis at the end of his life.

And to Mom, a 3 time cancer-survivor who got unlucky one fourth and last time. She challenged me every day for 35 years to become a better caregiver. RIP.
C.S.

To all my children, who made me see the joy in caregiving, and to my gran and mother, both cancer patients, who taught me valuable lessons about needing to care for myself first so I could be there for them when they needed me most. RIP.
A.S.

TABLE OF CONTENTS

ABOUT THE AUTHORS

Annabelle Stevens and Carolyn Stone are the authors of more than one hundred health and self-help guides. Annabelle works as a life coach and Carolyn has worked in consumer health publishing and continuing medical education for twenty years.

Praise for Coping With Caregiving:

5 stars - A must-read for people who might be caregivers in the near future
As someone who is not naturally inclined to be a caregiver, I found this book to be extremely helpful in preparing for the role of being the primary caregiver of my dad who is going through some pretty tough health issues right now. It helped me organize the myriad of thoughts that I couldn't quite wrap my head around when I was first thrust into the role of caregiver and derive a prioritized to-do list from them. For this reason alone, I would highly recommend this book to anyone who will be undertaking caregiving responsibilities soon and isn't feeling very confident about meeting the demands of this role.

But, if I didn't also mention the second reason why I think so highly of this book, I would be doing this book's potential readers a disservice.

To be an effective caregiver, not only do you need to know what to do in specific situations, you also need to know how to deal with the stress associated with being responsible for an ailing person's well-being. Stevens and Stone excel in this area by providing effective techniques that caregivers can use to manage their stress levels and not be overwhelmed by what is expected of them.

Are you going to be responsible for sick or disable person's care any time soon? Or have you found yourself flung into that role all of a sudden? If yes, you should definitely read this book.

5 stars – An excellent resource for all new caregivers

This is an excellent resource for anyone who suddenly finds themselves serving in the role of caregiver, to help prevent them from burning out. It deals with short-, medium- and long-term care issues with common sense and compassion for everyone involved.

I appreciated the experiences they share of their own backgrounds in caregiving. The chapter on the emotional side of caregiving was really excellent, with useful checklists of what to look out for. There were many useful suggestions for coping strategies if you are suffering from that negative emotion. I also really liked their list of the positive emotions involved with caregiving. It is not something I have seen too often in the research I have done since I suddenly became a caregiver recently.

Really glad I found this book. It is packed full of ideas and helps me to know I am not alone in this, that others, like the authors, have dealt with the same issues and got through it all. I also liked all of their handy suggestions on where to find more support and advice so I do not burn out or say something I shouldn't to the person I am caring for. The advice on how to say things in a way that will not make things more difficult worked the first time I tried it.

Best of all, I really appreciated their idea of me being the quarterback on the caregiving team. It makes me feel empowered, not a victim of circumstances, or pushed into things by doctors or other members of the family.

Highly recommended if you or a loved one are unlucky enough to get bad news at the doctor, and want to do all you can to work together towards a good outcome. Also excellent for anyone trying to care for a child or parent long-term. Burn out is very real but can be avoided if you know what to watch out for.

5 stars - A guide to care for others and care for yourself as well
This is a great guide to understanding the difficult sides of caregiving so they do not burn you out; depression, fatigue, sadness.

Helpful and thought provoking, encouraging Caregivers to take care of themselves, since that doesn't always occur for caregivers.

5 stars - Coping better with caregiving
For those teetering on burnout from either short- or long-term caregiving, you need support from family, friends, or professionals.

Having been a Professional for over 3 decades in Gerontology, having taken another position for a couple of decades, then retirement and travel, I was shocked to find myself having a screaming fit, caring for a friend with cancer. She has no living relatives, so for over 5 years I've cared for her in my home.

After so much stress, I looked for some guidance in this difficult service. I found this book to be a great road map back to getting myself cared for first so I can care for others effectively.

You are guided along a pathway to a new normal for yourself and the patient needing to be cared for as well.

5 stars - Excellent Resource for Caregivers
Coping with Caregiving is a comprehensive guide that provides information and action steps caregivers can take to help them deal with their responsibilities without the burnout that often accompanies taking care of someone in need.

The book addresses a range of caregiving situations, including caring for children and the newly disabled or ill, and stresses the importance of developing a care plan if and when you are ever put into the role of being a caregiver.

If you are a caregiver, or know someone who is, you will want to take a look at this book. It will save you time, energy, and possibly broken relationships.

It will definitely give you something to think about as you are performing your duties, to take better care of yourself so you can care better for others.

5 stars - Caregiver help is at hand
Great guide. Excellent insights. Really helped me see how important it was to care for myself first so I could do a better job caring for my mom.

DISCLAIMER

This guide is designed for general advice only. It is not a substitute for medical advice given by a qualified physician with respect to your own individual circumstances. You should never delay in seeking medical attention if you believe you are ill because of anything you might have read in this or any other health-related guide, website and so on.

Our authors provide updates of their titles annually to ensure that links and research are up to date. All content is correct and up to date at the time of going to press. However, due to the rapidly changing world of the Internet, authors cannot be held responsible for changes in third party websites and their content.

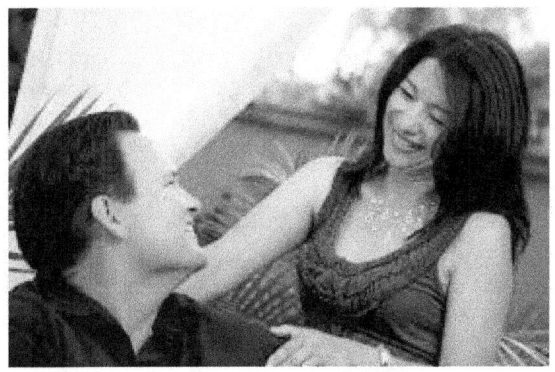

Introduction

Life can change in a split second. All it takes is an icy patch on the road or a drunk driver, a careless cyclist, a patch of wet leaves, or test results back from the doctor, and your life can be changed forever. Your loved one can suddenly become disabled, or told they have a serious illness, leaving them with a struggle you will naturally wish to help with, but are probably ill prepared to do so.

Our sister in law was barreled into by an impatient driver trying to run a red light. Our best friend was disabled in a car accident by a drunk driver who walked away without a scratch. Our step-father was knocked flat in at a busy street crossing by a bicycle messenger, and left bruised and bleeding, with a ulcer that began to bleed heavily.

Carolyn slipped on a patch of wet leaves while walking her beloved rescue dogs, and suddenly transformed from care-giver to in-need-of-care as all her friends and family rallied around to support her. Heart disease, acute kidney failure, and cancer touches the lives of so many these days, it might not be a question of IF but of WHEN one of your loved ones will be diagnosed with a severe illness that will require care.

Some people are born caregivers. Others have caregiving thrust upon them. We were both around 6 or 7 year old when we started to understand the whispers in our different households. Gallbladder. Ovaries. And the worst word of all, Cancer.

With over 30 years each of experience as caregivers for various family members and friends, we have created this guide with the new caregiver in mind, to help you care for yourself first so you can be there to care for others more effectively.

We all have loved ones in our lives with whom we share good times and bad. When something unfortunate happens to one or more of these special people, we can become devastated. In the blink of an eye, our lives have changed completely and unexpectedly.

The kinds of illnesses and accidents our loved one could experience may leave them disabled physically or mentally. Instead of independence, they find themselves relying on us for their day-to-day care. Both parties are left with a sense of loss and the sense of the situation being a stressful and difficult one, a burden.

The person who becomes the caregiver suddenly has a whole new set of challenges to deal with in addition to their already busy life. They might even end up as part of the "sandwich" generation, dealing with elderly parents or relatives and still raising children at home. Sometimes there will even be young children as a result of the fact that many people have put off having children until later in life.

In fact, this can even be a reason for them suddenly becoming a caregiver. Children can be born with birth defects to women of any age. Babies born prematurely pose a unique set of challenges. The caregiver might be in their forties already, and perhaps even be dealing with their own health issues already when they are unexpectedly thrust into the role of a caregiver for others.

The person who needs to be cared for during an illness or after an accident knows things have changed and does not want to be a burden. They can also be angry and resentful of having to be looked after by anyone. They can also be angry at the whole situation, asking, "Why me?" when in fact you might just as well ask, "Why NOT me?" Bad things happen to good people. It is how we handle this bad things that is the question.

Carolyn's grandmother was a world-class ballroom dancer who loved nothing better than to dance with her wonderful husband, until a drunk driver left both her legs and pelvis shatters, and one leg 4 inches longer than the other. She never danced again, but she was a pillar of her community, the mother most people never had, who never failed to light up every room she entered with her kindness and great sense of humor.

Our friend Doug, on the other hand, got a diagnosis of kidney cancer and refused all treatment. He died angry and almost alone, having driven just about everyone but Annabelle away with his fury over being ill.

Our friend Lee, a huge, burly man with a zest for expensive cigars and single-malt whisky, refused any painkillers and kept vowing to beat his pancreatic cancer even when he had dropped down to 85 pounds. His wife Evelyn could not even imagine all he went through in order to try to stay alive and be well again.

As people get older, their personalities can change, too, leaving already tense relationships and a difficult situation even more fraught with spoken and unspoken anger, aggression and hostility. At other times, the person we knew for years suddenly become withdrawn and unlike their former self. They might even start to fade away completely under the effects of an illness such as Alzheimer's disease, and need help with even the simplest task they were once able to do independently, such as walking and eating.

Children growing up with disabilities pose unique challenges at any age, and this can become more difficult over time if parents and family do not all pull together as a team to try to cope with the situations which will inevitably arise.

Even if we are just talking about a temporary illness, such as after surgery, several questions will go through the mind of the caregiver:

* Am I up to the task?

* What if I fail my loved one?

* Who can I turn to for help?

It is the last question in particular that can mean the difference between the family coping well and continuing to thrive, or one person in the family ending up with caregiver burnout.

Coping with the physical, mental, emotional and spiritual challenges of a loved one is a learning process, sometimes a steep one. When bad things first happen to good people, it can seem as if you are the only person in the world to whom this has ever happened. "Why me?" and "Why us?" are common questions that will often be asked once you are thrust into the role of a caregiver.

Just as with all things in life, you will never do things perfectly the first time you attempt them. However, over time, with practice, things can get easier, and you can become more skilled.

One of the most important parts of this process is the knowledge that you gain that will help you perform these tasks. From your initial fact finding, to mastery over your subject, can take weeks, months or years, but all the knowledge gathered over time will be put to good use.

Knowledge is power. Knowledge about the condition of your parent, or spouse or child will be key in doing a good job assisting them as their primary caregiver, but primary does not mean ONLY. You need to have a team in place so that you can get relief when you need it.

Everyone gets days off from their regular job. As the primary caregiver, it is no less important to have a practical schedule to get everything done and still have time to stay as stress free as possible considering the endless to-do list you will face.

As the old adage says, however, "A burden shared is a burden halved." You might want to think of yourself not as the primary caregiver, but as the quarterback or captain of the team, making what you hope will be the right plays.

This takes knowledge and experience, and an awareness of the strengths and weaknesses of everyone on the team, but it also means being aware that you actually have a team. You do not need to be the superstar and try to do everything yourself. What seems insurmountable at first can become manageable over time with the right support.

In the course of your caregiving, you may be forced to deal with physical challenges, mental challenges, or both.

A physical challenge refers to any bodily issues that prevent someone from taking care of themselves without assistance. It could be loss of function in a body part, impairment of some type such as damaged organs, or loss of a limb, that results in a diminished capacity for self-care and independence.

Mental challenges can occur from a birth defect, illness, or accident. For example, sustaining head injuries in an accident can leave many people with brain damage problems that range from memory loss, speech issues, or a lack of ability to exercise good judgment, to varying degrees of loss of physical function.

Some children are born with Down's syndrome, autism, or other mental conditions (though Down's does also have several physical aspects to it as well).

Then there are mental disorders, such as clinical depression. Chemical imbalances can result in schizophrenia, bipolar disorder, and much more, rendering the person incapable of fully looking after themselves. This can be true even if they are taking medications that alleviate their symptoms in some way.

Depression will often accompany severe illness, though researchers are not sure if it is cause or effect. For example, up to 75% of heart patients are likely to suffer from depression. Depression can be a severe complicating factor in the disease because it often causes people to not take good care of themselves or make the best decisions for their health and course of treatment.

Both mental and physical challenges represent a broad category of medical conditions. In each case, however, what happens is that someone other than the person affected has to take over as their caregiver, either temporarily or permanently, because the loved one cannot look after themselves.

In this guide, we will look at some of the common physical and mental challenges that our loved ones can face. We will examine ones that can happen at any age, and those that occur at particular stages of life and will generally persist for the duration of the person's life.

We will also discuss some of the main issues involved when you are thrust into crisis mode when a loved one has fallen ill, been injured, or is diagnosed with a health issue.

In all of these cases, you will need to learn quickly a number of things relevant to the immediate crisis so you can try to deal with it as effectively as possible, and also seek help from those who have more experience with the situation at hand.

If you loved one is suddenly taken ill or has an accident, for example, you will need to know:

*The diagnosis

*The prognosis (possible outcome)

*What care will be required, now, and in the future, and how long each stage of recovery will be estimated to take;

*How to deal with the loved one after the diagnosis, both physically and mentally

*How to deal with your own self-care issues over the short-, medium- and long term

*How to plan for the future given the possible outcome;

* Where to find reliable information and helpful support in reference to the medical condition, injury, or disability.

In this guide, we hope to offer the kind of advice and self-care strategies that will enable brand new caregivers to cope well without burning out. It is easy to do if you do not pace yourself. Sometimes caregiving might be for a short duration only, while at other times you could be looking not at days or weeks, but months or years.

The truth is that from the time you get word that you are going to been to help a loved one by serving as a caregiver, you need to view the situation as a marathon, not a sprint, and pace yourself so you are not run ragged.

The other truth that many people in society forget, even though it is common sense, is that you can't care for others effectively if you do not first take care of yourself and your own health.

Now that you know what to expect in this guide, let's be clear about what we will NOT be discussing. We will NOT be discussing any specific medical conditions because this guide is about caregivers, for caregivers by caregivers.

Every caregiving situation is different, just as every caregiver is different. We may have things in common as we deal with a mom with breast cancer or an uncle with lung cancer, or a cousin with dementia, but we are not going to give specifics about those or any other medical condition because that would be way beyond the scope of this book on caregiver burnout.

There is a lot of free information about those topics online, and in books. You can locate them using a good search engine like Google or searching at Amazon or Barnes and Noble. Our goal in writing this guide is to keep caregivers healthy no matter what kind of caregiver situation they are dealing with. Above all, we wish to help readers avoid many of the most common caregiving mistakes that can lead to burn out.

So now that we have gotten the preliminaries out of the way, in the next chapter, we will discuss dealing with the crisis when it first occurs, and how to cope when your loved one receives an unfavorable diagnosis.

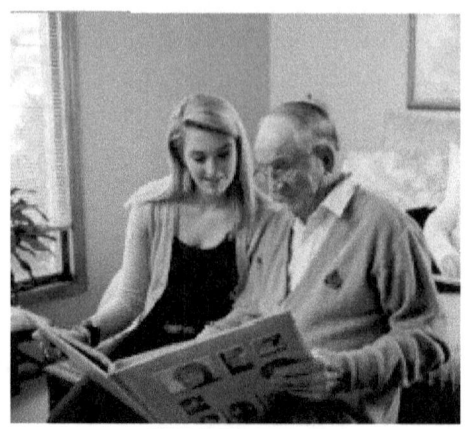

CHAPTER 1
DEALING WITH THE CRISIS

Things happen in life over which we have no control. Sometimes the events that occur are unpleasant and painful, and when a loved one suffers, it can be almost unbearable for us. When it results not in death, but in an injury or illness, most of us will want to help our loved one make it through the crisis, but often lack any knowledge of it and are thrust into 'crisis mode' and into 'diagnosis mode' (what it is) and 'prognosis mode' (what we can realistically expect the outcome to be).

For those of us who take out insurance policies for health, life, and short-term and long-term disability, we hope we will never have to use them, but understand that we are protected and covered if we ever do need to. When a crisis hits, however, this intellectual and practical grasp that bad things happen in life can often become overwhelmed by the emotions which arise when a loved one is injured or becomes sick.

Accidents happen all the time, often when we least expect it. One of our best friends from college, Cathy, and her closest family members were all rammed into by a drunk driver at 4AM just outside the airport they were driving to, on their way to catch a plane to go on vacation. They driver left them for dead and the only thing that saved them was a dog living in a house nearby who barked non-stop until his owner followed him down the dark country lane to the ditch the car had been rammed into.

Her father died, her mother had both her legs broken in three places, her brother's stomach ruptured, and she went head first through the windshield and woke up 3 weeks later to discover what had happened, and with facial injuries that required 4 years of plastic surgery to get her approaching something that even slightly resembled normal.

Her cousin in the car walked away without a scratch but was suddenly the caregiver for 3 critically ill people until she could get help from the more senior members of her family, who were all out of the country on their own vacations.

This is an extreme example, but also demonstrates that you can literally never know when you will be called upon to be a caregiver, and often you might not have any idea how long you will have to serve as one when a crisis emerges.

In many cases, you might also have to juggle work, other family commitments such as childcare, and more. Informing people of what is going on from the outset in order to get help and support is one of the best ways to ensure that you do get it, rather than adopt a 'wait and see' approach or try to shield others in the family from bad news. The latter tactic can often lead to you ending up as the caregiver with little or no help while others in the family leave you to deal with everything.

On the other hand, 'too many cooks spoil the broth'. However, not everyone leaves clear instructions about what to do in the event of an accident or severe illness. If there is no living will in place, for example, two or more children can end up disagreeing severely about how to care for mom or dad, end of life decisions, and so on, which can in turn mean that the injured or sick person's wishes are basically ignored.

An accident can change the lives of your loved one and the entire family in the blink of an eye. So too can illness, which is all around us. Dangerous infectious diseases in 2014 and 2015 have made headline news on numerous occasions, from whooping cough and Enterovirus to Ebola and now measles in February 2015.

No one is ever fully prepared for an unfavorable diagnosis from a doctor, who could tell us that our newborn child has Down's syndrome or has been born with a particular defect, such as a bad heart or only one kidney.

The doctor might also say that your loved one has heart disease, diabetes, even cancer, sending your loved one into a crisis mode as they have more tests to confirm the diagnosis and stage the cancer, that is, make an estimate of how far it has progressed in order to decide on the best treatment for the patient.

The National Comprehensive Cancer network has a number of cancer treatment protocols for a range of cancers that have been developed by over 20 of the leading cancer centers in the USA. As effective as they are, however, they are not a one-size fits all, and there are a number of choices that the patient will have to make, usually in conjunction with their cancer care team and also their loved ones.

When one of our colleagues told us that her husband had prostate cancer, we reviewed all the pros and cons of each treatment with them both in order to help him decide on a treatment he could live with in every sense of the term, and one she could live with too as his intimate partner, for whom maintaining a good sex life was also important.

That may sound like a strange priority, but the fact is that many people react to cancer in terror without weighing all their options. They often insist that the cancer be cut out ASAP, without ever even discussing the dangers of surgery, possible outcomes, and side effects, such as urinary incontinence and erectile dysfunction which can last 2 to 5 years, or perhaps even be permanent.

In some cases the crisis might be made worse by your loved one's reaction to the situation. They might try to shut you out, act angry, refuse to discuss options with you, and in fact, might refuse any treatment at all.

The way you deal with the crisis as a caregiver will often 'set the tone' for your situation as a caregiver, sowing the seeds of burnout before you ever even realize that it is a possible risk for you as a caregiver.

It is only natural to want to do SOMETHING when our loved ones need us and focus all our attention on them, but not eating or drinking, skipping meals, spending long hours in the hospital, and, dare we say it, not paying attention to hygiene in the hospital, can all leave you wide open to potential illness yourself.

Having working in the health field and been caregivers for years, we can tell you that hospitals are amongst the dirtiest places imaginable. They are also getting worse, with hospital-acquired infections, that is, sicknesses spread in hospitals, nursing homes and so on, all on the rise. One of our friends with a blood clot in his leg was actually sent home by the staff despite his condition because, they told him, they had had an outbreak of several infectious diseases in the hospital and were afraid he would only become sicker if they admitted him.

Even after the bad news about the accident or the diagnosis, once we know that our loved one will survive, it is the "what happens next" that scares most of us. This is partly a fear or realistic recognition that things are probably never going to be the same again, depending on the situation, and a natural fear of the unknown.

Until we have time to process what we have been told, absorb it, and perhaps start doing some research on what it all can mean, it is hard to grasp the scope of what we are possibly being asked to deal with or to do.

All we know at that point is that our life as we knew it is changing, and might even be gone forever. The question is, what exactly is going to be left in its place?

Of course, of the answer to that question will be unknown. Much will depend on the nature of the physical or mental challenges that our loved one has been confronted with. At times, we will become sorely tested in relation to our levels of patience, love, understanding, compassion and skills as a caregiver. We may have to learn new skills quickly, being given a 'crash course' in things we never imagined ourselves having to do.

When Carolyn's father-in-law was dying of liver cancer, for instance, she was suddenly called on to learn how to use a morphine pump to manage his level of pain as death approached. It was an important responsibility, because too little would leave him in pain and too much might hasten his death.

Learning all these new skills can be a positive experience if you know your loved one has a good chance of a full recovery, but it can be soul-destroying for some people if you know your loved one is terminal, because it all seems so futile.

But in our experience, most people concern themselves with living a good life, and if they ever stop to think about it, wanting a good death. Anything you as a caregiver can do to help them to a peaceful end is very worthwhile, for death is a natural part of life.

When confronted with a health crisis of any sort, the first thing we need to remember is that our loved one is still our loved one. Changes are occurring in your lives together all the time. An accident or illness will just be a more drastic one than most. Fundamentally they are the same person. We don't have to fear them or act guilty around them. What they need to see is that we still love them, "for better or worse," as the Christian marriage vows state.

This should also apply to anyone we cherish in our lives. If we value them, we will do our best to stand by them in their hour of need. However, it does not mean we should sacrifice our own health or career or things that are important to us because of the situation, because this can only lead to burnout and misery. Instead, we need to find balance so that everyone's needs in this new situation are being met.

However, this can be easier said than done. With small children in particular, it can be real challenge, especially if the child is born with a disability. A lot of parents have a picture of a perfect birth and delivery and a perfect child, only to end up with a premie on life support for 2 or 3 months.

When Annabelle's youngest nephew was born, his mother had the bitter disappointment of not being able to take him home when she went home from the hospital because he had such severe jaundice he needed to stay under the special lights designed to help relieve the condition.

She was even more disappointed when she could not feed the baby on the breast herself because he had weak mouth muscles and could not latch on. It was a race against time to feed him enough to flush all the toxins from his body before it was too late.

Luckily a breast pump and some Dr. Brown's bottles with the nipple holes enlarged for regular milk flow down the baby's throat saved the day. And because he was getting breast milk from a bottle, anyone could help feed him, so his mom could get the rest she needed after her emergency C-section. It also meant she could go back to work sooner and leave him with a childminder so she was not struggling financially as a new mom who had underestimated just how much everything would cost to care for a newborn, and how much the co-pays would be for all the special care the baby had needed when he was born.

One of the biggest challenges of being a caregiver is to give up on ideas of perfection or what "should" be happening. You will have to learn that good or very good can be good enough and that all any of us can ever do is try our best in any given situation.

We also must give up on any idea of "should" or "ought to" in relation to ourselves, and just deal with things as they arise, moment by moment. Otherwise you will be kicking against fate every step of the way, which is an exhausting state of mind that makes you tense, irritable, stressed and angry. It also means keeping on top of your finances, not letting bills and other essential paperwork slip, which can lead to unnecessary expenses such as late fees on your credit cards. It is bad enough to have to deal with health-related stress without also needing to deal with money-related stress.

As we know, mental stress can lead to physical stress and illness. With your loved one and perhaps others all relying on you, you can't afford to let yourself down, or you will be letting others down.

Therefore, be a good team member and give yourself time-outs when you need them. Keep everyone who needs to know informed about what is happening, which will give them a chance to help and support you. Accept whatever help they offer even if it is not appropriate, in order to avoid making them feel as if what they are attempting to offer isn't good enough. But do be honest as well-if the room is filling with flowers but you are not sure how you are going to pay the electric bill this month, tell a reliable family member or friend the situation to see if they can help.

Once you have been propelled into a crisis, or have an actual diagnosis, it will be time to dig more deeply into the condition and prognosis. Let's look at each of these in turn next.

THE CONDITION

Besides being at a loss for words when the doctor gives us the bad news about an illness or accident affecting our loved one either short-term, long-term, or for an unknown period of time, the shock will be difficult enough. Then there is the issue of trying to understand what it all means when you are already in an emotional daze.

We can be at a total loss to understand what our loved ones are suffering from. The change could be on the inside where we can't see it, compared to an accident, in which the change will be easily visible.

Learning all that we can about the condition that has caused the physical or mental condition can help us come to terms with the diagnosis. For example, if a loved one has been diagnosed with cancer or told that they will never walk again, it requires some research to fully understand the kind of cancer, its effects upon the body, treatment options available, and more. A diagnosis of MS can seem like the worst thing in the world, but now there are a range of treatments available that can help them live a normal life. In some cases, depending on the condition, there are even clinical trials run by medical institutions or pharmaceutical companies that they might be eligible for.

Carolyn's wonderful boss Ron went for colonoscopies regularly every year because his grandfather had died of colon cancer, but despite this, he was diagnosed with cancer-cancer of the appendix (appendiceal cancer), one of the rarest forms of cancer in the world. Apparently the scope can reach almost every place in the colon but two: the caecum (SEE-come), the join between the small intestine and the large intestine, and the appendix.

Some diligent research helped them discover that one of the world's leading experts on this form of cancer was in Pittsburgh, and so began a five year struggle with the disease, as he and his family regularly travelled back and forth from New York to Western Pennsylvania in search of a cure.

The cost would have been astronomical if it hadn't been for a clause in the insurance which Carolyn spotted that stated that if the treatment were not available through an in-network provider, the costs would be treated as in-network and covered fully apart from co-pays even if he had to go out of network.

We hope your loved one will not have anything so rare, but even if they do, you or another loved one doing research can help turn up a range of options you might otherwise not know ever existed.

The doctors will do their best to answer all your questions, but often they don't have a lot of time. In many cases, people also feel embarrassed about asking what is on their minds for fear of being thought stupid or judged in some way as not being caring enough or focusing on the right issues.

The more that you can learn about the physical or mental challenge your loved one is facing, the better able you will be to face caring for them. Go on the Internet and look up information, or read books in the library. Ask the doctor, nurse or other healthcare professional about your concerns.

It can be difficult to do the research when you are in the hospital by someone's bedside, but wireless connectivity can be a real lifeline, enabling you to look things up on your phone. Also ask if they have handouts, leaflets and so on that can help you and your loved one know more about what to expect. The departments at major hospitals will often have a standard set of patient handouts that you should read carefully. Make notes on them and/or note down any questions these materials might trigger as you and your loved one read them.

Online, locate discussion boards and forums related to the disease. You can often find very useful information from the perspective of both the patient and the caregiver, things the doctor might not know because he has not lived with the disease or the physical disability.

Being sure you have a reliable support network is one of the best ways to help yourself get through the days without feeling as though you are burning out. Three or four trusted friends or relatives can help you not just get through the days, but feel like you are happy again.

Your life may not be the way it was, but you can also start to approach a lifestyle that is a new kind of normal. We all dislike a change in our comfortable routine, but let's look at it this way. Think of the difference between when you were an infant, and your school days and then your work days as an adult. Then you will see that what you define as normal does change over time.

THE PROGNOSIS

The prognosis is the most likely outcome of the accident or illness. In most cases, it will be unknown, and that can be very frustrating and deeply worrying for all concerned. Even if recovery is guaranteed, for example, there is no certainty with reference to the time frame. When Carolyn broke her ankle in November 2013, she never imagined she would still be struggling with a weak-feeling joint in February 2015. Always the caregiver in her family, suddenly the tables were turned and hubby, Mom and the rest all had to start caring for her.

With cancer, the prognosis is definitely not certain. Even if a person has surgery to remove a tumor, chemotherapy, radiation and so on, there is still no guarantee that they will go into 'remission', that is, that the cancer seems to have been cured. There is always going to be the fear that it might come back, or that it might have spread microscopically through the bloodstream to another part of the body (metastasized-met-TAH-sta-sized).

The duration of care being so often unknown, new caregivers need to pace themselves in order to avoid burn out. After the adrenalin rush of dealing with the accident or diagnosis starts to wind down, it will be time to settle into a pattern of care which will hopefully not be at such a fevered pitch or so stressful. Again, it is going to be a marathon, not a sprint.

The amount of care, as in number of hours, and nature of the tasks, will also vary widely, and can therefore present the risk of burnout. Understanding that you can't do it ALL yourself and delegating can help prevent anyone in the caregiving team from burning out.

The amount of care that needs to be given will vary with the age of the loved one who has been affected, and with the condition. A mentally or physically challenged child will usually require more care on a daily basis than an adult might.

Or, a senior with Alzheimer's or another form of dementia might start to take up more and more of your time as their condition starts to worsen. Making sure you have a good support network in place and not trying to do it all yourself will be essential in both these cases if you are to avoid burnout.

In the case of a child being born with a disability, another issue to deal with is the feeling of guilt, especially on the part of the mother, that something they did or did not do contributed to the condition that now afflicts their child.

This is a normal reaction, but except in the cases of clearly irresponsible behavior such as drug taking, binge drinking, and/or risky sexual practices, will not be true. There are so many variables involved as a fetus develops that it is little short of a miracle how many babies are born healthy, rather than the other way around. Even if it is true, guilt will contribute nothing helpful to the situation, and only lead to burn out. Put the past in the past and deal with the present as it unfolds.

For adult sufferers of physical or mental challenges, the tables can be turned and their child now ends up caring for them, or for a sibling. Spouses also provide support to each other when challenges arise. Many can feel that "this is not what they signed up for," and it can be difficult to get personal needs met in this type of altered relationship. Again, a new normal needs to be worked out between spouses.

The Superman actor Christopher Reeve and his wife Dana were a good example of this. He broke his neck in a freak horse riding accident, yet they talked openly about the challenges of trying to maintain their marriage even though he was mostly paralyzed.

They discussed "outercourse" as a way to satisfy the sexual needs of both partners, and said that in some ways their new normal was better than their old way of living, much more intimate emotionally.

Sadly, he passed away from issues related to his condition, and she died not long after him from cancer. While we sympathize with their teenaged son and Reeve's adult children from his previous marriage, it was clear that they were extremely devoted as a couple, and so perhaps it worked out as they might have wished.

It is also clear through the foundation that Dana started and which the children are continuing that people respond to unexpected and very challenging events in different ways. Their success in helping children with similar accidents to walk again means that nothing is ever truly hopeless, and that new cures are emerging all the time.

Another issue many people think about and deal with in various ways is end of life issues. Some people prefer not to think about anything unpleasant; others want to know the worst so they can be ready for it, and hope for the best.

Depending on the mental state and personal characteristics of the person who is ill or injured, they have various options for treatment. The caregiver can often be left feeling helpless in the face of certain decisions, which might be made on the basis of emotions or logic, but not always through a balance of both. Regardless of which, to the patient concerned, not treating a disease can be seen as a viable option in some cases.

Annabelle's grandfather had just lost his wife when he was diagnosed with stomach cancer. As he said to her and her father, "I've lived a great life for 83 years, 65 of them with Gran. Now that she's gone, I have nothing to stay around for." He died of a stroke at home about 3 months later, never having had any treatment for the cancer.

This story is also an important one because he has served as his wife's caregiver for many years as she had aged and become diabetic. He illustrates the danger of looking after someone else to such an extent that they neglect their own health until it is too late.

Everyone responds to illness in different ways. Some are calm in the face of adversity. Some people make the decision that they are incurable. Others are so afraid of the unknown and the way life will be in the future that they delay seeking treatment until it is too late. Others do not seek treatment, or receive only minimal treatment, because they think their condition is some sort of judgment or test of their faith by God. We may not agree with their point of view. We might even think they are crazy. However, everyone does have the right to live, and die, with dignity, hard as that might be for any caregiver to accept.

In many cases, the treatment may not seem worth it for the little improvement in life span that can be gained compared with the side effects of the treatment. However, we always try to point out to people that while an additional two to six months of survival does not sound like much, and is by no means guaranteed, it does give everyone concerned some time to prepare for the end of life, getting their affairs in order and so on, if nothing else.

In many cases, they might be eligible for a clinical trial. If a trial meets with noted success in lengthening life, the treatment will often be made more widely available to others with the same condition. The person willing to undergo a clinical trial can certainly help others a great deal, even if his or her own lifespan is limited. A few years ago, there were no treatment options for kidney cancer, for example. Now there are several, thanks to those willing to enroll in and undergo the protocols for clinical trials.

One other thing we want to point out to caregivers and their loved ones is that doctors sometimes estimate incorrectly. We have seen many cases of people who were told they had a limited time left who survived long after the timeframe they were given. We have also seen people who were told they had months to live who went to sleep after they got the news, and never woke up again.

All of the examples we have given so far in this guide, and all the material that follows, is based on direct personal experience as caregivers over the years for a variety of family and friends. Looking back, we can honestly say that while every illness, injury, or health condition was different, the one thing that separated the success stories from the poor outcomes was determination and a good support team for the patient. In particular, it meant at least one person who served as caregiver who got the support and care they needed in order to stay the course and not burn out.

It is true that a person can have a great support team, but not determination. In this case, the caregiver may feel that all their efforts are worthless. Care and compassion are never worthless. However, you will have to realize that you are not the patient, and that while all your efforts are very praiseworthy, you might not get the result you are hoping for.

The best place to start to avoid a whole welter of emotions is with the facts. Once you have those, your understanding of the nature of the condition can often determine your plan for the future, however long or short that may be. It also means coming up with a care plan that meets the needs of your loved one and does not leave you as caregiver as a total wreck.

Any serious diagnosis can be a time of extreme stress, but with people counting on you, the best thing you can do is be as solid as a rock by learning as much as you can about the condition and then being helpful to others in providing information about care and needs, and finding the best strategies for a good outcome.

By all means pace yourself as you eat, drink, sleep, and do all of the essentials of your usual day. Get help with shopping, laundry, child care and so on. But also be sure to learn as much as you can so that you are well equipped to handle the care of your loved one yourself.

Respect their wishes, by all means, but also remember that you are the quarterback helping to make the key plays on the field. It will be up to you to implement the care plan to help move towards a favorable prognosis, if there is one, or a 'good death' if that is the prognosis.

In the next chapter, let's look at the topic of drawing up a practical care plan that can help the patient recover or maintain a high quality of life, without you suffering from caregiver burnout.

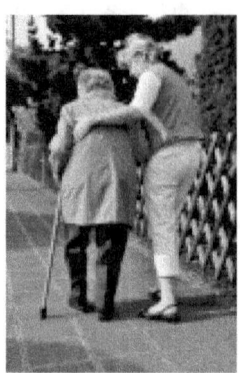

CHAPTER 2
DEVELOPING A CARE PLAN

Most of us start out each day with a to-do list. Once you are faced with the prospect of becoming a caregiver, your to-do list will change. You will need to switch directions and goals in order to cope with the needs of a loved one who suffers with a physical or mental challenge.

In this case, though, you will have to work in conjunction with your loved one, if they are capable of making their own decisions, and their doctors. Beginning to formulate the steps involved in devising a practical care plan can be confusing and may involve some false starts.

It will certainly involve searching for resources to help your loved one with their own particular condition. Even in small communities, there can be more help available than you may think if you spend some time putting out feelers and asking for guidance and advice.

Begin with the closest possible resources to your home, and work your way out from there to help build a network that can act as a safety net for you and your loved one now and in the future.

Possible resources for a loved one's care are:

* Churches

* Charitable foundations (Make a Wish, Ronald McDonald House, etc.)

* Organizations and charities dedicated to a particular illness

* Hospitals

* The Federal government

* Pharmaceutical companies and their charitable divisions

* Medical schools and their researchers

* Hospitals.

Putting together the plan might need to begin long before the loved one ever comes home from the hospital. For example, if they are recovering after an accident and you know they will be in a wheelchair for some time, you might want to make adaptations to your current living situation sooner rather than later when they have already arrived home.

If you are renting your living space, you might consider trying to find a new place better suited to your loved one's needs, such as a building with an elevator instead of stairs.

This can be particularly true in the case of an older patient, who might no longer be able to live in their own home by themselves. In this case, it might be a whole family decision as to where the parent is best off, with which child, or perhaps in an assistant living facility or a rehabilitation center or nursing home, depending on the degree of care they might need.

Churches offer their support for members in need and loved ones of a fellow member. Their support comes in the form of prayers, cooked meals, house sitting, and transportation if it is needed and can be arranged. Some church groups have adaptive vehicles such as minivans that can safely carry a person in a wheelchair. In large cities, there will also be accessibility programs that can help you and your loved one get around to doctor appointments and so on if you do not own a car or vehicle that they can get into easily.

Often it is a case of asking for what you need and finding out what is possible. The trouble with many caregivers is that they don't ask for help because they do not want to bother anyone and think that they need to learn how to manage by themselves.

As the great Renaissance poet John Donne wrote: "No man is an island, entire unto himself." None of us live in isolation. None of us can be self-sufficient. We all need to work together as a team.

Some players on the team might expend more effort than others, but at least put them to the test to see if they rise to the occasion. People generally tend to pull together when they discover that a person they know has a problem, and they are willing to help.

The best way to take them up on this offer is to tell them what needs doing and then let them work out their own way to help. No one can micromanage other people. Give up all notions of "perfect" or how you would do it better if you had the time. Learn to delegate and then once the chore is done, cross it off the to-do list until next time.

Charitable organizations work to assist families with information and support for a loved one. The Make a Wish Foundation grants wishes to terminally ill children. Ronald McDonald House provides a place for family to stay when a child is in need of medical care far from their home.

Other organizations offer services and financial help to qualified individuals, with the criteria varying depending on the organization and the case.

Organizations dedicated to a loved one's particular mental or physical challenge help families better understand what is going on with their loved one. The large organizations will raise funds, offer free or inexpensive resources, and help educate people about the particular condition. Checking with such an organization can yield a bounty of information and where to get help, both from the organization itself, and people who work with it as advocates, experienced caregivers, and more.

Hospitals employ dedicated nurses and doctors who care for patients just like your loved one. Before leaving the hospital, it is important to ask all of the questions you have about care and treatment. Using state of the art equipment, hospitals provide medicines and rehabilitation to people who need it, but these treatment regimens can only be effective if the patient follows the guidelines set forth.

On discharge from the hospital, for example, they will probably be given a number of prescriptions to be filled, and all the instructions must be followed. This will be particularly true in the case of pain killers and other addictive medicines, and also for medicines being used to treat potentially life-threatening conditions, such as high blood pressure, heart disease and diabetes.

You may want to set a clock or an email reminder that will text your cellphone or the loved one's to keep them on schedule with all of their medications.

You might also wish to invest in a daily or weekly pill box, depending on how much medication needs to be taken. These items have pre-marked containers so that all they would have to do is reach in to get their dose at the correct time. They have different configurations, with a number of compartments per week or day, such as four compartments if a person had to take a certain medicine four times each day. Then once a week, you would load up the containers.

While a lot of people think not much help can be had given the current state of the economy, you would be surprised at how much help there is. Drug programs offered by pharmaceutical companies and other groups can help people get the medications they need, but might not be able to afford.

Social services can also assist caregivers in applying for a loved one's benefits such as social security and disability. If the loved one has been working, there are different rules for short-term disability and long term disability. Be sure you know the rules and regulations for each.

The Federal government can apprise a caregiver about the rights of their loved one according to the Americans with Disabilities Act. You will need to do your research and be sure you have all the relevant data from doctors that will be needed in order to file a successful claim. Be warned that it can take time and involve a good deal of frustration to get your loved one's entitlements. In some cases, you might want to consider hiring a lawyer who specifically handles disability benefit claims. Some people have waited up to four years to finally get accepted on disability and begin receiving the money to which they are entitled.

Many of us should have an emergency fund set aside for unexpected expenses, but very few of us have four years' worth of living expenses set aside (see the Money Matters series at Eternal Spiral Books for more on this topic).

Caregiving is an emotional and physical issue. It can also be a financial issue as well, especially if the illness or accident results in a reduced income, which can cause a real shock to the family finances.

Let's look at the financial aspect of your caregiving plan in a bit more detail.

THE FINANCIAL ASPECTS OF CAREGIVING

There can be a lot to do when it comes to handling the financial aspects of a loved one's life after they have been diagnosed with an illness or had an accident.

This will mainly apply to an adult parent or sibling who needs to move to be closer to you, the caregiver. This might involve selling their home if they can no longer live alone. Getting their financial affairs in order is important when it comes to finding the resources needed to help with their care.

The same is true if the ill or injured person is your spouse. Things can become particularly difficult if they were the main wage earner in the family. In this case, it can be hard to try to keep things stable with a lot less income. If you were also working, it can be difficult to try to take on the role of caregiver when you also have a career to consider.

Finances also come into play when it is your child who suffers from physical or mental challenges. Their care can include lengthy hospital stays, special equipment at home, and even home healthcare visits. All of this costs money and can quickly max out your insurance and savings account if you don't have a plan in place that makes the most of the assistance available to you.

In some cases, you also need to get advance approval from the insurance company for visits to specialists, equipment and more.

Your loved one may end up needing financial support for many years, or perhaps the rest of their life. Depending on the illness or nature of the injury, this can be either a short time or many years. It can also involve intermittent care, or intensive care.

Even more important to the outcome than finances, though, can be the support of loved ones, the emotional connections and bonds that are tested severely during these times. In some cases, events such as these can bring people closer. In other cases it can tear families apart. Let's look at the importance of the emotional support of loved ones.

THE EMOTIONAL SUPPORT OF LOVED ONES

A person needs their family more than ever when they suffer from a physical or mental challenge. It is not that they want to rely on your help, but without it they would be almost totally at the mercy of strangers and institutions.

Taking care of an elderly parent or a family member with an illness is not something we think will ever happen, but with people living longer than ever before, this is occurring more and more frequently as the first wave of the Baby Boomers has reached retirement age and many have chronic illnesses with which they must cope. Some people

CAROLYN STONE AND ANNABELLE STEVENS

are more emotionally equipped to deal with certain issues than others.

The best way to deal with caregiving issues is to try to approach them on a whole-family basis. For family members who are far away, help could take the form of helping financially to care for the loved one.

No family member wants to feel as though they are facing such a huge responsibility all alone. Typically the care of a loved one falls on one or two members of the family. This situation can cause resentment and an overburdening of a small number of caregivers. On the other hand, a lot people trying to get involved can be a case of too many cooks spoiling the broth.

In the case of married couples where one of the pair is suffering, the other spouse is the primary caregiver. The children may help if they are old enough, and also the siblings and parents of the loved one. No matter what, it will often be a difficult time for everyone in the immediate family. Any offers of help should be accepted, if possible, but there is a fine line between help and interference.

For example, a well-meaning parent or sibling of the ill or injured person may express their views and opinions of what is being done in a very critical way, without stopping to think that their views might be hurtful or uninformed. No one knows what it is like to nurse a loved one with cancer until it happens to them. No one is ever prepared for these situations either, and all anyone can ever do is to try to cope with whatever arises.

The loved one does have a choice about their own care and treatment. They might also need a lot of emotional support and reassurance that they are doing well. They might also decide not to opt for treatment at all.

Dealing with other members of the family can be difficult enough. Reaching agreement with the ill or injured person can be complex, if not impossible, at times. Let's look at this issue in more depth in our next chapter.

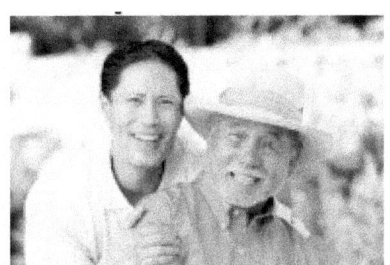

CHAPTER 3
DEALING WITH A LOVED ONE INDIVIDUALLY

It is hard to know exactly what another person feels unless you have personally experienced the same issues that they have. Even then, everyone experiences suffering in a different way; therefore, we can only guess what they will be feeling mentally and physically, and try to support them as best we can.

When a loved one experiences a condition that leaves them with a physical or mental challenge, it is devastating for us, and can be for them as well if they are aware that their life has changed.

A child who is born with a disability may have a very different perspective on their situation compared with an adult who recalls all the things they used to be able to do before their illness or accident. They can feel pressure to get back to normal as quickly as possible, or even go into some sort of denial and pretend that things are just fine.

It is an understandable response. Their life has changed from what they knew or wanted. Now they are adjusting to a new way of life with someone else in seemingly in charge; the doctor, the caregiver, or even the disease itself can be resented as taking over their life.

Denial that there is even something wrong is another approach, but it can lead to disaster. Denial can cause the ill or injured person to not seek the treatment that they must have, or make their illness or injury worse.

When we experience a temporary illness such as a head cold or a broken leg, we look to our family to pitch in around the home. We don't concern ourselves too much about it because while we do not want to be a burden, we are assured that sooner or later the cold will go away or the leg will heal. When we are better again, we will do our fair share around the home once more. We will even happily be a caregiver to others when these events occur.

With a terminal illness, accidental injury, or diagnosis of a mental condition, the situation is quite different. It can either be short or long-term, but with no one knowing how long. With a terminal illness, we know we are not going to get better and be able to help our loved ones one day.

With a physical disability, we might be forced into the realization that it will not go away no matter how much we wish that it would. With a mental disability, some people are more aware than others of their condition, and this can cause them stress, anxiety, embarrassment, and even anger and acting out.

Every person is different, and every day is different in the course of your new life with them, one you are trying to build to resemble the old one as much as possible in most cases.

In other cases, however, we have seen people completely change their lives, often for the better, as a result of their own illness or that of a loved one. For example, a workaholic husband might suddenly wake up to the fact of his not being there for his family when his wife suddenly develops cancer.

Another person might look at herself and her overweight husband who has just had a massive heart attack and decide that they are going to lose the weight and start taking better care of themselves in order to be alive long enough to raise their toddlers to college age and independence.

In many cases, however, people either don't know what to do, or refuse to follow instructions, either not willing to give up control, or through depression and despair.

Denial can affect both the loved one and the caregiver. Both wish that things could be different, but the facts have to be faced sooner rather than later. Getting a loved one to deal with the reality of their situation is not an easy task.

For children who are ill or injured, their understanding of the condition falls on the parents. Children are resilient and will respond well in most cases to the new normal that their parents need to try to help create for them. If you act as though their condition is not a big worry, so will they. A child will accept who they are if they get a strong sense of self-worth from their parents. The physical or mental challenge may set them back a bit, but it doesn't put them out completely in most cases.

There are professionals who can help, depending on the condition, and you should also enlist the aid of the staff at the school your child attends, and even educate the other children in their class and perhaps also the parents.

Remember that not all disabilities are visible, and even ones that seem simple can be dangerous. Think of the increase in the number of peanut and egg allergies among children, which can cause them to go into shock and die within minutes. The recent case of a teenage couple who kissed after one of them had eaten something with peanut hours before shows that everyone involved should be made aware of a child's condition and how potentially serious it can be.

Many people are reluctant to talk about illness, but a little knowledge can help save a life. One of our friends had a teacher at school who everyone gossiped about, saying they thought he was often drunk in class. After a biology lesson in which they had learned about diabetes, she started to suspect that he wasn't drunk, but ill. Her guess proved correct when she was in school late one evening and found him unconscious in the school corridor.

She got him to respond and made him drink a sugary soda she had with her, and also eat a candy bar while she called an ambulance. The paramedics who arrived told her that he probably would have gone into a diabetic coma if she hadn't acted so quickly, and might even have died.

People who live alone do not tend to take as much care of themselves as people in intimate relationships. We can see this from the studies conducted on life expectancy and health conditions in married or partnered people versus single people.

So while it is true that for an adult loved one, reality can be difficult, it is also true that the support of others, especially their partner, can mean a world of difference.

A lot of what the ill or injured person is going through can be the result of misplaced pride. Just the thought of someone else being burdened with their care can turn into disgust and self-loathing. How can anyone love someone who is crippled or a shadow of their former self?

The Christian marriage vows state that you will love your spouse for better or worse, for richer or poorer, in sickness and in health. In most cases, people truly mean those words. They may not always show it or be a perfect caregiver, but most people who care about their loved one will be willing to try their best.

Understanding the details of the medical condition can often relieve a lot of fears and anxiety. In many cases, what they think is going to happen might be far worse that what actually does.

In some cases, the risk of losing the loved one can result in a better relationship for both people because it leads to more understanding of feelings, both physical and emotional. For example, a person with a missing limb may need to learn to walk all over again or write with their other hand.

People with missing limbs often feel phantom pain in the missing limb. Knowing that lets you know they are imagining things when they feel phantom pain, but that it is a real symptom of their condition. Through understanding, you can cope with the condition and be more supportive than a partner who does not get as actively involved in their partner's treatment.

A loved one may resist the urge to ask for help in the beginning. That can cause issues for the caregiver who doesn't know what to do for their loved one. They will feel helpless, as if they are not doing enough.

When you understand what to do to help with their care, you assist them in subtle ways, whether they specifically ask for your help or not. This can help the caregiver feel empowered and the loved one will appreciate it even if they do not say so. It is all a question of striking a balance and trying to be there to help and support, but without being too intrusive.

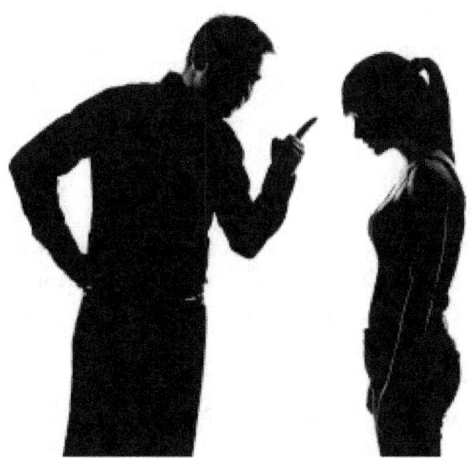

TOUGH LOVE

However, sometimes it does pay to intrude. In certain cases, intervention is the best way to deal with certain issues that the loved one will be going through.

For example, in a case where a loved one can wallow far too long in their denial and depression, and want to give up on life, it will be time to intervene in a number of ways. At times they may not even seem to be the same person that you loved. They will get angry, push you away, and be rude at every turn.

A frazzled caregiver who did not take steps to deal with this in a firm manner from the start would be a wreck within a week. Your loved one is clearly upset and angry, but they are also testing you. They cope by pushing your patience to see how much you can stand. It is a test of love, right or wrong, consciously or unconsciously.

Some caregivers feel guilt and give in to their loved one's every demand and take all the insults that are doled out without a word of complaint. However, this is clearly not an acceptable kind of relationship in the long term; it is abusive and will only escalate if it is not halted from the outset.

Permitting this kind of behavior allows the caregiver to give them message that it is all right for their boundaries to be violated. This sort of behavior has to stop on the part of both parties, or the cycle of guilt and anger will continue and the loved one won't ever get better.

Practicing tough love is the solution, although not a pleasant one. We use this tactic on our teenagers when they misbehave and get out of hand, and others who are, for example, in the throes of an addiction and require an intervention.

To jolt them out of their self-centered actions, it is time to take the hard line. It is because we love them that we try to re-establish boundaries and get the relationship onto a more even keel, using tough love to state the facts of the case in an unemotional way and call upon the aggressor to see their pattern of behavior and make the decision as to whether they are willing to correct it or not.

For children, our guilt can cause behavioral problems for them. A toddler with a disability will still behave the same as any other toddler. They will try your patience as they learn the boundaries of acceptable behavior. The trouble is that if you make too many allowances for them because of their disability, they can start to get very spoiled and unruly.

Discipline teaches them that they are the same as anyone else and gives them a sense of values. Even a challenged child needs discipline, though they may not always respond to it in the way that you might hope.

You may have to come up with creative ways to teach them right from wrong if the challenge is mental, but the discipline still needs to be there. Time-outs, chores they don't enjoy doing, and so on, can all work depending on the age of the child and the extent of their disability. Whatever punishment is given should also be in relation to the offense.

Above all, everyone in the family needs to be consistent. It is no good trying to discipline any child if mom or dad turns out to be a soft touch and do not back you up.

Playing favorites with them is also not a good idea. If you have two boys and a girl, regardless of which child has the disability, everyone should have an equal number of chores. The chores will only differ in length and difficulty depending on age and physical or mental status.

In some cases, being a good caregiver can also be about picking your battles and letting some things slide, instead of being a control freak who wants to have everything be perfect. For example, if your loved one does not want to be washed by you for several days, give them the means to do so each day, providing basin, soap and washcloth; do not make it into a battleground.

If your parent with Alzheimer's wants to shout and curse at you, leave the room or pretend not to hear. Let them know that their tactics won't work to ruffle you and that you have better things to do than stand there and be insulted.

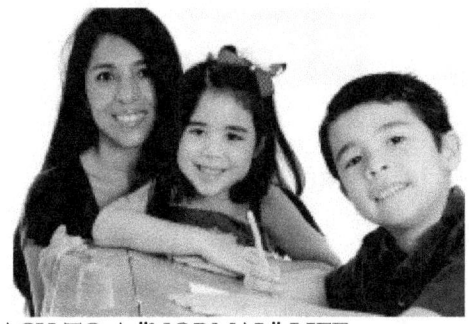

GETTING BACK TO A "NORMAL" LIFE

For a long time, your loved one might want to see only you or other family members and not your wider circle of friends and community. To enjoy their lives again fully, they will need to re-establish those relationships. For people that don't understand what has happened, it is necessary to see the person and reconnect, and explain things to them in simple terms.

People fear the unknown, so you will find that sometimes even people whom you considered to be very close friends will have a hard time coping with you and your loved one once they have become ill or injured.

In other cases, people are not sure what to do, and don't wish to intrude, so they stay away, and this can make them seem distant or disinterested. Out of sight can often mean out of mind for some people as well.

It is also sadly true that people tend to rally around after the initial illness or accident, but fall off after a while once things seem to be getting better. This is the time, however, when the two of you could use the most help, when you are coming to terms with your new normal. It would also give you time to relax a little bit now that you are no longer in crisis mode.

As a caregiver, go with your loved one to visit friends. Talk openly with them about the condition and answer any questions they have. They will begin to get comfortable again with your loved one, which is what everyone needs.

They can also get comfortable with you in your new role, and hopefully be willing to help fill in from time to time so that your loved one does not get tired of seeing the same old faces and you don't feel like a shut in.

If you are dealing with an older loved one or a child, do not make the house into some sort of extended sick room with everything revolving around caregiving. Try to have as normal a family life as possible, with all sorts of people coming over to visit and you hosting potlucks and so on.

You may not be able to be the world's greatest hostess because you have so much to deal with, but if you can't get out to the party too often, have the party come to you.

Try to exercise and get some time to yourself every day, even if it means trading babysitting during the day with a neighbor to keep an eye on your sleeping mother or child, with babysitting for their children in the evening once your spouse gets home so they can get a date night.

Speaking of date nights, it can be hard to try to have a normal marriage when everything is revolving around caregiving in the household, but it is important to try, even if it just means going into your room with a takeout meal and a bottle of wine to spend some quality time together. A baby alarm works well for both parents and children to alert you if anyone needs anything in another room.

An experienced home health worker can also come in from time to time to help you and your spouse get out of the house and spend quality time together.

Cooking and cleaning will not be as easy as they were when you had more free time, but don't be afraid to ask for help or even hire someone to do these chores. This will be especially important if you are trying to hold down a job and be the main caregiver at the same time.

Juggling a lot is never easy, but dealing with illness and caregiving issues can be physically, emotionally and financially draining if you don't all work together as a team to help focus on getting the best care possible for the person who needs it while still taking good care of yourself.

Let's look at this topic in more detail in our next chapter.

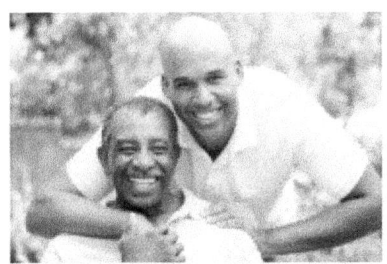

CHAPTER 4
TAKING CARE OF THE CAREGIVER

Caregivers are a special group of people who give selflessly of their time to care for others. Some people are natural caregivers, and others are thrust into the situation when the need arises due to a loved one needing help.

Not everyone is cut out to be a caregiver, and some will take a more hands-on role than others. It is sad to say, but some people know they can't cope, or are not committed enough to the other person to want to cope, and the relationship ends. That is certainly no reflection on the sick or injured person, but rather on the person who decides not to deal with the situation in a compassionate way.

For most caregivers, though, they go to the opposite extreme, giving two hundred percent if they can. One thing that caregivers have in common is the tendency to neglect their own needs; in particular, health needs, as a result of caring for others.

They become so focused on their loved one and what they need that they forget about their own needs. Even if they realize that rest is warranted, they push the thought to the back of their minds because they feel that they can't get away, or that they will do it tomorrow.

As we know, when we put off doing things, tomorrow often never comes. Therefore, it is crucial for the caregiver to try to pace themselves and do things that nourish body, mind and soul each day. In this way, they will be in much less danger of caregiver burnout.

Let's look now at the most important issue with respect to caregivers, taking care of their own health even as they take care of the medical needs of another.

TAKING CARE OF YOUR OWN HEALTH

Caregivers have to take the time to take care of themselves or else the whole caregiver system will fall apart. Someone else is depending on you. If you can't get out of bed in the morning, that person won't get any care at all unless you have outsider help on call, which most people don't because they do not have a back-up plan, feel they can't afford it, don't want a stranger in the home, or think that they should be able to handle it all by themselves.

Their reasons may be any and all of these things combined, but it can result in putting an unnecessary burden on their own backs. Even if the loved one you care for needs around the clock care, there are moments when they can fend for themselves. We all sleep at one time or another, so a caregiver could get their own rest and relaxation during that time.

Many people hurl into chores and housework and just make themselves more stressed. If you don't want to or can't afford to delegate healthcare, then delegate housekeeping; is a lot cheaper and can help you stay in balance.

Get older children to help with chores and don't feel as though it is charity if your church group or other well-meaning people offer help. Chances are you have helped others in the past, so now it is your turn to be aided when you need it most.

Take a half an hour or so to relax, read, and then another thirty minutes to exercise. If you can't leave home, set up a small home gym with dumbbells and a portable DVD player and then rent a group of exercise DVDs from Netflix. Change up your routine so you don't get bored and try a variety of activities to see which suit you best, and work on whatever trouble spots you might want to tone and trim.

It does not all have to be vigorous aerobics either. You can work your muscles without needing to worry about injury with high-impact routines (which could be a disaster if you could not then fulfill your caregiver duties). Belly dancing and zumba are two popular choices.

A good relaxing, but also deep muscle exercise is yoga. Yoga relaxes the body and the mind through a series of stretches and poses. In those moments of quiet exercise, you can recharge your cells and renew your spirit as well.

You should also plan on going for a walk every day if you can, with your loved one, if possible, or on your own if you can manage to leave them alone or with a sitter. If you can't get away outdoors, you might want to invest in a treadmill and jump on it every chance you get.

Even ten minutes at a time will add up over the course of a day. Just be careful that you don't injure yourself, as they require some getting used to and many injuries are caused by people not paying attention and falling. If you can't afford a treadmill or have no room for it, think about a stationary bike. You might also jog in place every chance you get.

Good nutrition in the foods you eat will also be key to staying well while you care for others. Nourishing your body means putting high quality food into it, not junk food. Protein and a range of nutrients keep your body supplied with all the building blocks for a healthy body and immune system.

Your immune system in particular needs to be cared for with vitamin C, and the effects of stress reduced with vitamin B products. You might want to take a multivitamin to help supplement your nutrients if you are eating on the go a lot (see our guide on this subject for more information).

Antioxidants are also essential for counteracting the effects of free radicals on your health. Free radicals occur naturally in our bodies, but can also be caused by smoking and an unhealthy lifestyle. Green tea, chocolate and blueberries are all great sources of antioxidants and can act as great pick-me-ups during your busy days. (See our guide on antioxidants and free radicals for more information on this topic.)

Staying healthy thwarts those cold and flu germs that attack in fall and winter. You will also probably want to get a flu shot so that you can try to avoid the flu, which might lay you low. In this case, you would not be able to care for your loved one. The flu coming into the home might also end up worsening your loved one's condition, which you will want to avoid at all costs.

You will also need to get enough sleep to help maintain your health and wellness. Eight hours of high quality sleep are needed to help the body rest and repair itself. If you are getting short-changed, you will soon start to feel the effects, getting run down and not able to perform all of your important caregiving functions.

It may seem impossible to get enough sleep, especially if you have a newborn at home with health concerns, but take it in turns with your spouse if you can, or sleep when the loved one sleeps. (For more information on the importance of sleep for your health and weight, see Carolyn's guide on the subject.)

Exercising, eating right and getting enough sleep are the most important aspects that are under your control when it comes to maintaining your health. Make sure that you take time for yourself no matter how much other people are relying on you, because if you don't, you could end up not being there for the very people you are trying so hard to help.

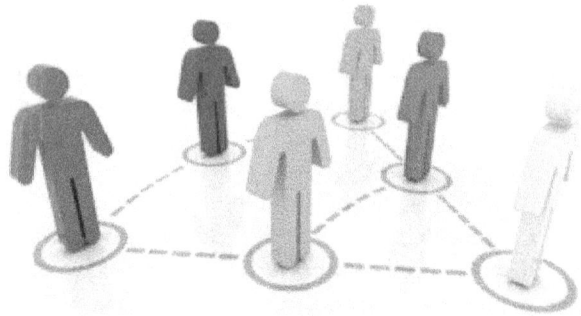

CREATING A SUPPORT SYSTEM

Everyone needs a break, and that includes caregivers who are caring for a loved one full time. It doesn't mean that you love your family member any less because you need a night out without them. If they were healthy, we wouldn't spend every waking moment with them; we would spend time with friends, and so on. Therefore, try to stay close to your friends even if you are crunched for time. They could prove a valuable mood lifter during some of your more trying times.

And often however badly off we think we might be, hearing another person's story can make us put things into perspective and see that we aren't so badly off after all.

Find a support system. Even if you can handle the care of your loved one, it would be easier if there were others you could talk to that understood your feelings. Frustration can set in rather quickly when there is no outlet for your feelings. That frustration can be felt by your loved one, who may assume that you feel that they are being a burden to you.

Frustration is a form of anger. It usually starts with an assumption that things ought to be a certain way; however, that assumption comes from your own mind. In that case, if you let go of the idea of ought to or should, the frustration will not arise. You will be able to deal with whatever arises moment by moment in a flexible, not tense and stressed way.

Your life is not forfeited over completely because you are caring for a loved one. Use close family members and local services to help find the time to get out and be with others.

Elder care and child care services give your loved one a place to go for the day so that you can have some time alone or with others. Just getting out of the home can seem to be a hassle, but change is a great way to elevate mood and keep people stimulated.

You will also want to attend support groups, and should go regularly at the start of your role as a caregiver, when you will need emotional support the most. Try to go often even after you have seemingly got into the groove of caregiving and have started to establish your new normal.

The support groups can be face-to-face meetings or online. Support groups help the caregiver understand their feelings and offer a chance to vent if they have to. Also, a support groups allow for meetings with kindred spirits who also care for a loved one and may have a lot of useful knowledge to impart when you are still in the steep learning curve stage of what to expect and how to deal with certain illnesses.

Couples who have young children can often be in a difficult position if one of their parents becomes ill. They must provide for their own children and spouses while still handling things for their parent. One method of support for them would be taking turns with other family members with respect to care, or doing it during the week, especially if the loved one is living with them, but getting weekends off.

Everyone in the family should try to pitch in together to meet the needs of the loved one and their full-time caregiver. This can also take the form of financial assistance for home health workers and so on.

The question of what each family member can contribute can sometimes be a confusing one. Some families may be well off financially, while others may have more free time, or more experience with caregiving. In this case, a balance needs to be struck so that everyone offers what they can best contribute.

Many options are open to the caregiver for alternative care for their loved ones. The objective is to make the process of care easier for the caregiver to handle, while not neglecting their families or themselves in the process.

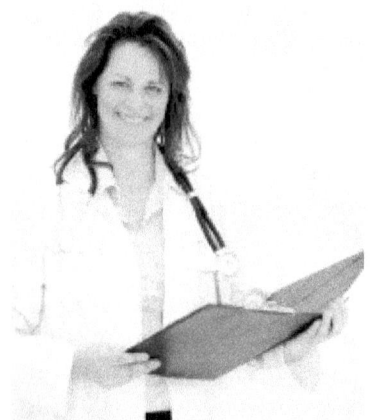

GETTING PROFESSIONAL HELP

Many people are reluctant to ask for professional help because it costs money and can seem intrusive. However, if it can stop caregiver burnout, it is a great reason to give yourself a day off once a week if you can.

A lot of home healthcare worker agencies can charge a lot of money for referrals and so on, but you might wish to determine if any local nurse or other healthcare worker would be interested in giving you a hand for a few hours a week at a reasonable rate. Many nurses in our area, for example, only work 12 days of the month in 12 hour shifts, leaving 18 of their days free.

Use as many free resources as you can in terms of information, and days covered for hospitalization, rehabilitation, nursing home care and so on. Then see what is still needed and how to fill in the gaps. Even having one day off a month is better than none.

You need to avoid caregiver burnout no matter how long you serve in the role of caregiver, for a short or long period. Your loved one may be on a clear track to getting better slowly but surely, or they might have a less than favorable prognosis. In the latter case, you will need to deal with end-of-life decisions.

These can be difficult at the best of times, but even harder if you are frazzled and burned out. Asking for professional help can not only assist you in dealing with a situation which most people feel is way beyond them; it can also leave you confident that the best decisions are being made without any overly emotional involvement getting in the way of taking action.

With all of the health information freely available on the Internet these days, don't discount the professional advice that you can find online from reputable health websites. Study all your options for caregiving, treatments, and strategies for coping with a physically or mentally challenged loved one, but don't neglect your own health in the process. Use the support groups to give you practical advice and information. Above all, use them as a valve to let off steam in order to help you deal with the emotional aspects of caregiving. Let's look at this topic in the next chapter.

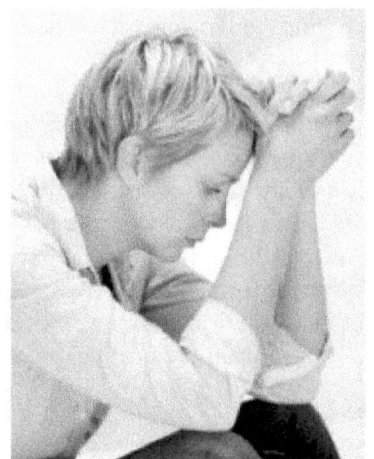

CHAPTER 5
COPING WITH YOUR EMOTIONS

We have touched on your emotion and that of your loved in in the course of this guide as we have discussed the practical aspects of making the transition into caregiving as an important part of your daily life. The longer the caregiving goes on, however, the more likely it is that negative patterns and negative emotions can start to creep in, persist, and contribute to caregiver burn out.

There are many emotional aspects involved with caregiving, from positive feelings about your new role, to negative ones that can creep into our minds even in the best situations. Caregiving is just a new level of responsibility in what is already a pretty packed life, and a new source of stress as we go about our busy day. In this chapter we will discuss some of the positive and negative emotions often encountered by caregivers, and strategies for dealing with these emotions in a healthy way in order to avoid caregiver burnout.

We will also discuss how to spot signs of stress, and stress relief and relaxation techniques to try to keep you in balance on your caregiving journey.

Positive Emotions Involved with Caregiving

Contrary to popular belief, there are actually many positive emotions involved with caregiving. Focusing on them even when the going gets tough can be one way to help maintain balance in your life and avoid caregiver burnout. Common positive emotions include:

+Love, Tenderness, Affection
+A Sense of Purpose
+A Sense of Doing Something Worthwhile with Your Life
+Pride in Your Accomplishments

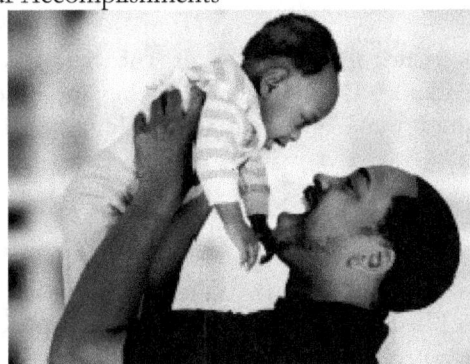

Love, Tenderness, Affection

Caregivers care. You will be caring for your loved one, and might experience a whole new level of love, tenderness and affection as you do so. You will be happy they are with you and might even enjoy spending more time with them, even if the nature of that time might have changed.

If it has changed, you will need to work together on achieving a new normal, but focusing on the love will help you focus on what matters most, preserving the relationship.

If your relationship was undergoing a tricky phase before the incident that resulted in you becoming a caregiver, you might start to feel a whole new sense of affection for your loved one. You might also feel guilt or grief over 'not loving the person enough' or over loss of your former life together. (See more on guilt and grief below.)

On the other hand, your new normal can be a positive, a fresh start for you both if the prognosis is good. It can also be seen as a way to experience closure if the prognosis is not good, making the most of the time you do have with each other by cherishing your loved one for as long as you are together.

7bac8d1f-d0e7-46b4-9cb0-8571299f7b1d.006.jpeg

A Sense of Purpose

Some people have a very full life, career, family, hobbies. Others drift from job to job and just live day to day. Caregiving can suddenly stop the drift and give you a sense of purpose and focus as you care for your loved one. Some people might run away from the challenge of caregiving, but others rise to the challenge and suddenly discover all the things that they are capable of.

One of our friends tells the story of when she was diagnosed with a serious heart condition. Her doctor was talking about her after care when she finally left the hospital and went home. He said, "My best advice is to get a dog."

"A dog?" she said in surprise. "Why?"

"Because no matter how lousy you feel, to the point where you will not want to get out of bed some days, that dog will be depending on you. It will stop you feeling sorry for yourself, love you unconditionally, and help you get the heart healthy exercise you will need every day to stay well and live a longer life."

The doctor was suggesting that caregiving for the dog would give her a sense of purpose in her life. And in fact, studies have shown that nearly 75% of people who have a heart condition also suffer from depression. Owning a pet can enhance mood, and so can regular exercise. Nearly 20 years later, Evelyn is alive and well, healthy, and an ardent dog rescuer. She was able to transform her own illness into caring for others and in doing so, discovered a whole new purpose in her life.

In the course of getting her first dog, she went to the local pound, where she met a man who looked as shabby as any homeless person she had ever seen. He was known as Matt the Cat, and as hard as it was to believe by looking at him, he had once been one of the most successful lawyers in the country, wealthy, ambitious, with the perfect life and seemingly the perfect marriage.

One day he found a new born kitten in his front yard. He determined to nurse it to health himself. From that one tiny kitten he hand reared with an eyedropper and milk around the clock, he began to help more and more animals, to the point where he stopped taking high profile cases and his wife left him because he was no longer the top executive she had married.

He turned his country home into an animal shelter and placed pens on every available spot of land on the property so he could rescue more.

In Matt's case, caring for one kitten has led to tens of thousands of rescues and finding good homes for them all, even though he was the last person anyone could ever imagine 'having gone to the dogs', as he jokes. His example might be extreme, but as he says, even his worst days in animal rescue are better than his best days as a lawyer.

These two stories also bring up an important point, that caregiving for a pet can be a challenge. It can be just as stressful and demanding as caring for any human loved one. Pets give us unconditional love, and rely on us as their humans to make the right decisions for them. Since they do not live as long as we do, caring for a pet such as a cat or dog will usually involve about 15 years of commitment and end of life decisions at some stage.

Many humans can go through all of the intense emotions and caregiver burnout in relation to pets in a similar manner to those experienced by carers for human care recipients, and should diminish their feelings, or allow others to dismiss what they are going through as no big deal because it is 'just a pet '.

A Sense of Doing Something Worthwhile with Your Life

As we have said, some people drift from job to job and interest to interest without a clear sense of purpose or any goals. Caregiving can give them the sense that they are doing something important and worthwhile in their life. They will of course need to balance their own needs with those of the loved one they are caring for, but it can be really powerful to see positive results in your caregiving efforts and make you want to do more.

We have already told you about Evelyn and Matt and their sudden transformation into animal rescuers. Another of our friends, a top Wall Street executive, needed to care for her husband for many months after he was in a severe car accident.

Once he was back on his feet, she enrolled in nursing school and is now head nurse in one of the best hospitals in her area. As good as she felt about wheeling and dealing and making money, nothing could compare to the satisfaction of helping people heal.

Pride in Your Accomplishments

Caregiving can be the toughest job you will ever love. It will challenge you every day, presenting you with new skills to learn and obstacles to overcome. You will probably learn a great deal about a particular medical condition and gain hands on experience of treating it, what works, and what doesn't.

You will get help and advice from doctors, nurses, and people in support groups. As you gain experience, you will be able to help them in return. You will become an expert in some cases, possibly even knowing more than a lot of health professionals thanks to your in depth research and observations on what works and what doesn't when you are caring for your loved one.

Caregiving often reveals sides of ourselves we never knew we had, ones we can take pride in as we add to our skills and gain in confidence. That pride can help push you through the tough times and even empower you to take on new challenges, like Lori giving up her seven figure salary to become a full time, qualified nurse.

One of our friends' daughters helped care for her father during the nearly five years that he lived with cancer before he finally passed away. His battle was over, but hers was just beginning. She was so proud of all she had learned and achieved that she did a premed science conversion course to bring herself up to speed on all the science requirements she would need in order to switch from liberal arts to being accepted to medical school. She passed with flying colors, got accepted to one of the top schools, and is now a fine GP and researcher.

We hope that you too will experience these more positive emotional aspects of caregiving regularly, but the truth is that coping with caregiving can be like riding on an emotional rollercoaster with no way to stop it, and often no end to the ride in sight. This is because in many cases, we do not know how long it will take for our loved one to recover, or in some cases if they will even recover.

The daily grind of any job can also get us down, but caregiving offers a unique set of challenges. Not being aware of emotional stressors that can trigger caregiver burnout can be one of the easiest ways to become burned out.

In the next section, we will deal with some of the most common emotional states caregivers experience when looking after their loved one. Note that these emotions are often experienced by the care recipient as well, further complicating your caregiving situation.

The main thing to remember is that you cannot serve as an effective caregiver if you are burned out. It is not selfish to put your emotional needs first, because no one else will be able to get their needs met if you are hanging on by a thread. Therefore, make sure you tend to your own negative emotions first with effective strategies, to put yourself in a better position to be able to care for others.

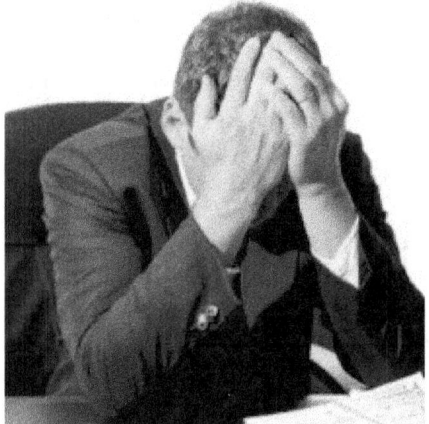

NEGATIVE EMOTIONS ASSOCIATED WITH CAREGIVING

It is normal to feel negative from time to time in general, but it does not usually cause so much stress that you feel as though you are overwhelmed and can't go on.

However, once you become a caregiver, the negative emotions can start to outweigh the positive. In this case, you need to be vigilant about caregiver burnout.

The most common negative emotions caregivers experience are:

*Worry and Anxiety
*Sadness and Depression
*Anger, Frustration, Lack of Patience, and Irritability
*Guilt
*Grief and Bereavement

On the following pages, we will outline the most common signs and symptoms of each emotion, so you know what to look for. We will also list tried and tested coping strategies in case you do discover you are suffering from one or more of them.

Worry and Anxiety

It is natural to be concerned about your loved one and how your new caregiving situation will affect your household and your relationship, but too much worry can prevent you from dealing with your situation effectively.

Signs You are Experiencing Worry and Anxiety

*Worrying a lot about everything, or about one thing over and over again.

*Feeling stressed out, edgy, or overwhelmed.

*Sweating the small stuff in a way you would not usually do. .

*Dwelling on things you would normally brush off as unimportant.

*Feeling short of breath.

*Feeling physically tense and uptight.

*Indulging in emotional eating whenever you experience a change in mood.

*Feeling negative all the time, as if something bad is going to happen, or only imagining the worst in each situation.

Strategies for Coping with Worry and Anxiety

*Prepare yourself as a caregiver by reading books or searching on the Internet for information about your loved one's condition.

*Make a list of all the things you are worried about. Just writing them down can often bring some degree of relief.

*Use your list as an action plan. Once you have identified the issues, try to come up with steps to deal with each one effectively.

*Talk to other caregivers by joining a support group, chat rooms on the Internet, or linking up with other caregivers through advocacy groups. Find general ones, or condition specific ones.

*Schedule time to do things you enjoy.

*Schedule time for breaks.

*Make time for exercise, to relieve tension and improve your mood.

*If feeling panicked, take some slow, deep breaths.

*Relieve anxious thoughts by using guided imagery, yoga, meditation, or something that relaxes you. See the section on relaxation later in this chapter.

* If your worries start to paralyze you from taking action, consider seeking professional help.

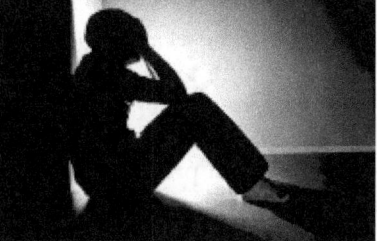

Sadness and Depression

It is natural to feel sad from time to time, especially if your loved one is suffering and your life has changed drastically as a result of suddenly being thrust into the role of a caregiver. Sadness that never seems to lift, however, could be a sign of something more serious, such as depression. Depression is now the second most common cause of disability in the world, after vision and hearing loss. With your loved one counting on you, you cannot afford to become disabled by depression.

Signs You are Experiencing Sadness and Depression

*Feeling down all the time, often with no particular reason you can pinpoint.

*Feeling tearful or emotional.

*Bad appetite, obvious weight loss.

*Overeating or eating unhealthy comfort foods, with obvious weight gain.

*Sleeping too much.

*Sleeping too little, or suffering from insomnia

*Erratic sleep patterns=trouble falling asleep, trouble staying asleep.

*Loss of interest or enjoyment in your usual activities.

*Feeling like you want to give up.

*Thoughts of suicide, 'ending it all.'

Strategies for Coping with Sadness and Depression

*Exercise to improve energy level and mood.

*Focus on good things in your life.

*Eat small meals packed with protein, and steer clear of foods high in carbohydrates, such as sugary or starchy foods.

*Deal effectively with sleep deprivation and insomnia so it does not become a vicious cycle.

*Talk about your feelings to a close friend or family member.

*Join a support group online or in person.

*Seek the help of a mental health professional if you feel no relief from your sadness after trying several strategies. Also be sure to seek help if you have thoughts related to self-harm or suicide.

The National Suicide Prevention hotline in the USA is at:
1-800-273-TALK
1-800-273-8255

You can also get help and advice on this and a range of topics from the Samaritans 1-212-673-3000

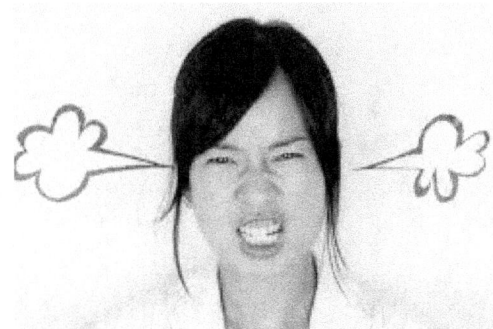

Anger, Frustration, Lack of Patience, and Irritability

When you first become a caregiver, you will usually run on adrenaline, doing what you have to do in order to help your loved one and just get through each day. But over time, your new role can start to tire you, leaving you prone to negative emotions such as anger, frustration, a loss of patience, and irritability.

In particular, if you are caring for an older relative who has a dementing illness, you can grow more and more short-tempered. You will be giving care around the clock or worrying about their affairs even if they are in an assisted living facility, but will see few results and no sort of progress for your efforts.

Signs You are Experiencing Anger, Frustration, Lack of Patience, and Irritability

*Feeling annoyed easily.

*Feeling irritable over small things.

*Feeling short tempered, especially if your loved one keeps doing the same thing over and over, such as with dementia patients or children with learning difficulties asking the same questions repeatedly even when you have just given them the answer.

*Feeling like you are going around in circles and getting nowhere.

*Feeling like your life is not living up to your expectations.

*Being verbally aggressive with others.

*Being physically aggressive with objects-hitting, pounding, slamming doors, breaking things.

Strategies for Coping with Anger, Frustration, Lack of Patience, and Irritability

*Try to live moment by moment, with no expectations of success, progress, or the way things should be.

*Try not to sweat the small stuff.

*Do not suppress your anger. Find ways to let off steam in a harmless way, such as exercise, thumping a pillow, taking a walk around the block, and so on.

*Do not sound off about your feelings without thinking about the consequences. You do not have to suppress your anger, but you also do not need to say everything that is on your mind.

*If you do feel you have to share a negative emotion, try to do so in a positive way. For example, you could begin by saying, "You know how much I value our relationship, so I want to share something with you that has been on my mind."

* If you do get angry, look at your own mind to trace the cause of the anger. Is it justified? Or is it possible that you might not have all the facts? Also try to look at the situation from the other person's point of view before flying off the handle.

* Transform your thoughts from negative to positive using whatever strategies work for you, such as guided imagery or relaxation exercises. See more on relaxation techniques below.

*If you try all these strategies and still have a hard time dealing with your anger, consider an anger management class or support group.

Guilt

Guilt is the sensation of having let oneself down, or someone else down in some way. It can be based on something that you have actually done and regret, or on something you imagine you could have done differently, or should not have done. Guilt might have some basis in fact, or none at all.

Regardless of the real or imagined reasons for the guilt, guilt can damage relationships and prevent you from being an effective caregiver. It is sometimes used as motivation to do things you might not otherwise do because you are forcing yourself to, or because you are being manipulated into feeling guilty by others, including your loved one. Beware of guilt to help keep your stress levels down and avoid caregiver burnout.

Signs You are Experiencing Guilt

*Feeling like you have done something wrong, or that you are responsible in some way for what happened.

*Feeling like you are not doing enough for your loved one.

*Feeling like you should not enjoy yourself, especially in relation to things you used to do together, because your loved one is no longer able to.

*Feeling guilty about any negative thoughts and feelings you may experience in relation to your new situation as caregiver.

*Feeling like you have neglected other friends or family members due to caregiving.

Effective Coping Strategies for Guilt

*Guilt can come from feeling bad about thinking "unacceptable" thoughts. Try not label thoughts or emotions as good or bad, acceptable or unacceptable. They just ARE. Accept them as a passing thought or fleeting emotion and move on.

*If you have done something you feel has injured someone else, do not jump through hoops to try to make up for it. Instead, admit your fault, apologize, and ask for forgiveness.

*Do not be too hard on yourself. No one is perfect and mistakes happen.

*Actions can have unexpected consequences. If this happens, remember that it is your good intentions that count.

*Express guilty thoughts and feelings to a friend, support group, or mental health professional. Just talking about them and not suppressing them can often make the guilty thoughts lose their power over your mind.

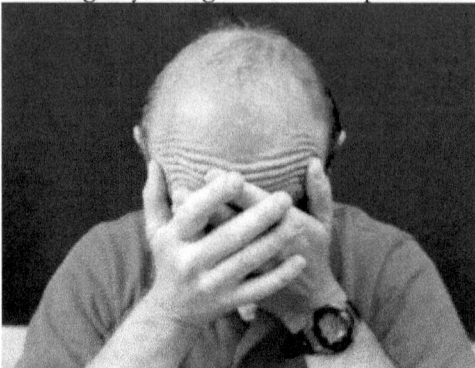

Grief and Bereavement

Grief and bereavement can come about for many reasons. In the case of suddenly being thrust into a caregiving role, you might feel grief and a deep sense of loss when you compare your former life to your present one. You might also start to experience grief over the loss of a loved one even when they are still with you, such as when you are caring for a loved one with a dementing illness, or a terminal one. In these cases, the outcome will not be a positive one, leading to a sense of frustration, anger, futility, and grief.

Grief can also be triggered by thoughts of what might have been, but of course, we have no way of knowing this; it is mere speculation or fantasy, and as such can be very unhelpful if you wish to avoid too many downs in the emotional rollercoaster that many people experience in the course of their caregiving.

Living in the now rather than the past or the future can be one of the best ways to avoid grief and bereavement. Cultivate an attitude of gratitude by being grateful for the little things and treasuring them.

Also do not be afraid to talk about end of life issues. It is a difficult subject a lot of us wish to avoid, but in many cases, death helps define life and give it meaning.

Signs You are Experiencing Grief and Bereavement

*Experiencing emotional pain associated with the loss of anything that is an important part of your life.

*Feeling sad about changes in the person you love.

*Feeling upset about your current relationship with him/her, and comparing it with what you had in the past and finding it lacking

*Being disappointed about lost hopes, dreams, and plans for the future.

*Feeling powerless about changes in your life and relationships.

*Feeling upset about changes in your work/professional life as a result of being thrust into a caregiving role.

*Dwelling on what could have been, rather than what IS.

Strategies for Coping with Grief

*Allow yourself to grieve for changes in your life and plans for the future.

*Try to focus more on the positive things in your life, rather than the things you have lost.

*Do not isolate yourself from family and friends.

*Try to keep to your regular routine as much as possible.

*Know that feelings of grief and loss are normal and that, given time, the acute pain will subside.

*If you are experiencing negative feelings, know that in time they will diminish, leaving happier memories in their place as you achieve closure and move on to a new chapter in your life.

*Express your feelings to the patient or others close to you as appropriate.

*Avoid feeling guilt over any sense of loss or relief that your loved one is no longer suffering.

*Talk to a mental health professional or join a support group.

Caregiving is not usually a sprint, but a marathon. The finish line in some cases will be recovery for your loved one, but as our population lives longer than ever before, the finish line might also be a complete lapse into dementia and eventual death, or death from an illness or injury. In the case of a child born with learning difficulties or birth defects, it might be their death, or you trying to leave them as well off as possible before you and your spouse pass away.

Like all marathon runners, you need to run a smart race, pacing yourself so you do not give in to exhaustion. The practical aspects of caregiving can be time consuming and demanding, leading to continual levels of stress. Add chaotic emotions to the mix and your course can become a bumpy one. But you can smooth the path and avoid caregiver burnout by learning a few general strategies for dealing with emotions as they arise in a healthy way. Let's look at a few of these next.

Dealing with Your Emotional Needs in a Healthy Way

Whenever a loved one is sick, we naturally want to do as much as we can to help them. But as time goes on, it can be very easy to feel like our needs do not matter compared to those of our loved one.

Nothing could be further from the truth. Only by remaining strong can you maintain your own physical and emotional wellbeing. It is not selfish but sensible to pace yourself and be honest about your needs and desires, and get them met in a healthy way.

If you are calm, relaxed and fulfilled, instead of constantly on edge and feeling as though you are 'running on empty', you will be a far more effective caregiver than someone barely hanging on by a thread.

Do Not Suppress Your Feelings

Start by getting rid of any idea that there are good and bad feelings. Think of them as a cloud appearing, going across the sky, and vanishing below the other horizon. If you do not dwell on your feelings, they do not have the power to affect you negatively in the long term. Recognize them, register them and any possible reason why you might feel that way, and then let them go.

If you do feel like you can't shake a certain negative thought, confide in someone in your support network. Often just talking about the feeling can help it vanish.

Suppression and dwelling with how you should or shouldn't feel can only make things worse. Stop dealing with 'should' and just deal with what IS, moment by moment.

Give Yourself Outlets

Everyone needs a break from their work in order to rest, relax and rejuvenate. The biggest problem with caregiving is that it rarely has regular hours. Far from being a nine to five, it can be around the clock, depending on the nature of the condition and the independence or otherwise of the care recipient.

You need to schedule regular breaks to avoid caregiver burnout. Even when you are 'on duty', you should also schedule short breaks for yourself to provide outlets for yourself so your stress levels do not get too high.

Regular breaks can prevent you from feeling overwhelmed and suffering from caregiver burnout. Only by caring for yourself will you be able to care for others effectively.

Plan breaks for exercise, entertainment, and time to relax, unwind and decompress. If you loved to take a hot bath before you became a caregiver, this is the last thing you should sacrifice except in the very short term, such as when you first become a caregiver. Reintroduce them into your routine again once things start to get more in balance. Also be sure to include outside activities in your day, such as a trip to the park or local coffee shop to meet a friend. Remember, you are a caregiver, not a prisoner, and that being a caregiver is a lifestyle choice, not a life sentence with no hope of parole.

Strategies for Making Time for Yourself

*Don't feel guilty about wanting or needing time away from your duties as a caregiver.

*Know that it is okay and necessary for you to have some time for yourself.

*Make a list of people whom you trust to care for the patient during your absence. Then ask someone for help at a specific time, on a specific day. Even if they can't commit to a regular care slot each week, they can certainly fill in a 30 minute gap here and there for you to get a break so you can avoid caregiver burnout.

*If you don't have anyone in your family or social circle who can help, you can obtain a volunteer or hire someone for a short time. You may be able to locate such people through churches, community groups, local agencies.

*Allow yourself time to focus on you and you will feel refreshed and not burned out when it is time to take up your caregiving duties once more.

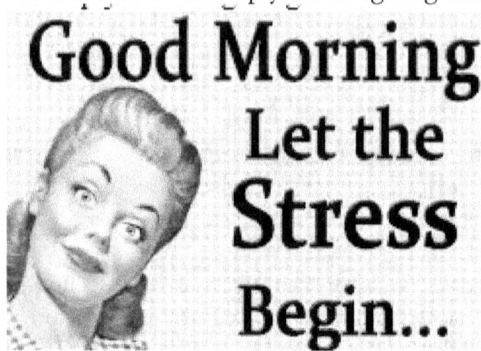

Managing Stress

Everyone experiences stress, from the child at school taking a test, to a worker having to give a presentation to senior staff, to the person who receives a phone call saying there has been an accident. It is how we manage the stress on our caregiver journey that can make all the difference between healthy caregiving and caregiver burnout.

Stress can manifest itself in a number of ways, including mental, emotional, physical and behavioral ways.

Here are a few of the signs of stress to watch out for:

MENTAL

*Finding it hard to concentrate

*Having trouble remembering things

*Feeling foggy

*Having a hard time making decisions

*worrying all the time

*Seeing only the negative side of things

EMOTIONAL

*Mood swings, often with no clear cause

*Irritability, a bad temper

*Feeling agitated all the time, finding it hard to relax and let go of things

*Feeling out of control or overwhelmed

*Feeling lonely, even when surrounded by a lot of people

*Feeling sad all the time, or depressed

PHYSICAL

*Aches and pains, such as headache and backache

*Diarrhea or constipation

*Nausea, dizziness, vomiting

*Changes in appetite, such as none, or an uncontrollable one

*Chest pain, rapid heartbeat, irregular heartbeat

*Loss of interest in intimacy

*Frequent colds or other illnesses

*Sleeping too much or too little, or insomnia

BEHAVIORAL

*Spending a lot of time alone

*Putting off important tasks or chores

*Showing little or no interest in things that were once important to you,

work, family gatherings, community get together such as faith based gatherings, etc.

*Using alcohol, cigarettes, caffeine or drugs to get you through the days and nights

*Suddenly developing repetitive habits, such as nail biting, pacing, tapping, twitching your crossed leg, etc.

*Feeling like you are just not yourself and behaving in untypical ways

Strategies to Help Relieve Stress

Here are just a few suggestions to try. Use the ones that work for you, and the ones you have time for throughout your caregiving day.

*Go for a walk around the block.

*Spend time in nature, such as taking a stroll through the park.

*Call a good friend and chat for a few minutes.

*Sweat out tension with a good workout. Even if you cannot get to the gym, have a few workout DVDs on hand. And 4 ten minute sessions can be just as effective as one forty minute one.

*Write in your caregiving journal.

*Take a long bath.

*Light scented candles.

*Savor a warm cup of herbal tea such as chamomile or peppermint.

*Watch something funny for a few minutes, such as on YouTube.

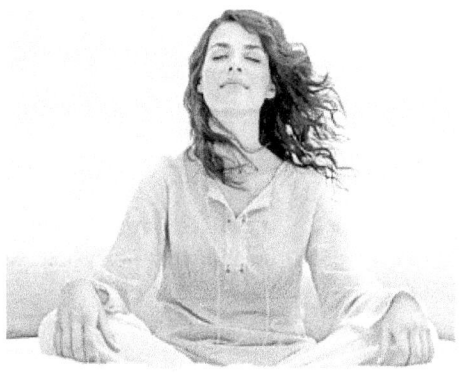

Use Relaxation Techniques as Needed

Stress is a part of modern life, but it can start to take a physical toll on our body, mind and spirit if we do not take steps to minimize its impact upon us so it does not get the better of us.

There are a number of relaxation techniques that you can use any time to take your simmering emotions off the boil and calm down. Here are a few suggestions:

Diaphragmatic Breathing

Breathe deeply from your belly feeling all your muscles and ribs expand and contract as you take slow, deep, long breaths.

Visualization and Guided Imagery

Some people have a set visual image they go back to time and time again, a 'happy place' they can picture in their mind that will help them instantly relax and feel less stress. Others might use guided imagery, going to a place or a certain process in order to feel more peaceful and at ease. They might use an audio tape or mp3 to take them through the guided imagery or repeat the same words to themselves as they imagine themselves going on a journey to their happy place.

You can rely on your imagination, or you can look online or in magazines for inspiration. Take yourself away for a few moments to your favorite place. Use images from the Internet or pictures you have taken to help you. But do not escape too often, as too much guide imagery can cause you feel discontent with your present situation. Balance your breath, and the ideal with the real, to see what a difference it could make to your stress levels.

Meditation

Meditation can help you calm your thoughts and gain new perspectives on things that are troubling you. Go to a quiet place, sit comfortable, and focus on your breath, noticing how you breathe in and out, and how each breath can cleanse and calm you and prepare you to face the rest of your day. You can find many lessons online which can help you learn to improve your skills, learn to deal with stress, and more.

Body Consciousness

Take five to ten minutes to lie down alone quietly in a comfortable place. Set an alarm if you are worried about falling asleep. Once you are lying comfortably in your chosen location, start to pay attention to each part of your body, starting with the toes and working you way up to the top of your head. Notice any tightness, tension, tingling, or aches and pains as you work your way up. Pay attention to your breathing as well, aiming for long and deep, not short and shallow. Back pain or neck pain, headaches and indigestion can all be signs of stress to watch out for.

At the end of your scan, imagine a powerful golden light bathes your sore spots. After allowing yourself to feel warmed by this healing energy, thank your body for helping you get through the day and do all the important tasks you have to perform. Respect your body and be a friend to it, and it will be a friend to you.

Avoid abusing your body through bad habits. Let's look at a few of these next.

Unhealthy Coping Strategies to Beware Of

Sometimes people respond to illness or adversity through unhealthy coping strategies, both the care recipient and the caregiver. Unhealthy coping strategies can include smoking too many cigarettes, drinking too much alcohol, consuming too much caffeine, or eating unhealthy foods or too much 'comfort food' which might be high in carbohydrates and fat. To avoid temptation, it is best to avoid having these items in the house. In this way, you will not automatically reach for them when the going gets tough in your caregiving. By eating healthily and avoiding mood altering substances, you will be in better control of your emotional rollercoaster and less likely to suffer from caregiver burnout.

If kind helpers keep bringing you meals you would not normally eat, thank them, portion it up into small portions, and freeze the food for future consumption as a little treat. If they keep bringing food that is unhealthy, tell them subtly about the kinds of things you and your loved one generally eat as part of a healthy lifestyle.

If they still persist, give them a couple of recipe cards for your family favorites. Tell them to try them and let you know how they turn out. If they still persist after a lot of hints, you can always fib and say you or your loved one is allergic to a certain ingredient. That will usually stop people from giving you unwanted food and also avoid any questions, hurt feelings, or comments like, "Go on, have a little, it won't hurt."

Some people eat a lot of sugary foods full of empty calories, or foods high in carbohydrates. They only give a temporary burst of energy, but will then leave you with a 'carb hangover', tired, moody, hungry, or sleepy. Stay alert by eating fresh, natural foods, and avoid heavily processed foods containing white sugar or white flour.

Caffeine is a pervasive drug in our society, but it can leave you prey to mood swings and too much can give you a buzz that will set you on edge and make you less in charge of your emotions.

Recent studies on caregiver stress have shown a few keys to success. They include not having too many money worries, having a good support network, and the caregiver not being too old and in good health themselves. The research also shows that social participation versus isolation seems to be a key factor in caregiver stress versus success. By avoiding unhealthy behaviors and habits and staying connected with others, you can maintain your own health and help avoid caregiver burnout.

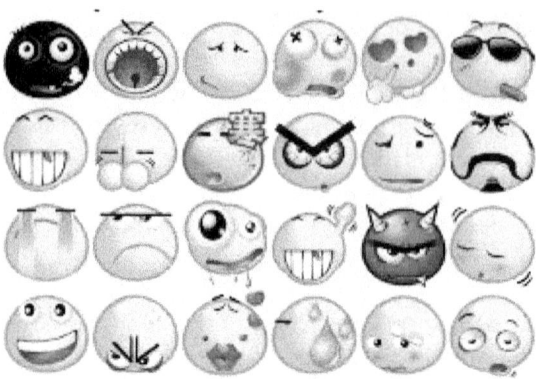

Expressing Your Feelings-To Speak or Not to Speak?

It is common to spend so much of your energy supporting the patient that you end up ignoring, holding back, or failing to recognize your own feelings about the situation. Continuously ignoring your own feelings can be very dangerous. Feelings can build up until you become so stressed that you can no longer handle the situation.

For this reason, it is extremely important for you to identify and address the feelings that you are having, and then decide whether or not it is wise to share what you are feeling with your loved one. Here are some specific, appropriate ways to express and cope with your emotions.

*Identify what it is that you are feeling and allow yourself to accept the emotions as a natural emotional response to the stressful but rewarding job of caregiving.

*Use a range of proven strategies to deal with the emotional aspects of caregiving such as we have discussed above in relation to a particular emotion.

*Do not bottle up your feelings, but try to express them in a healthy way.

*Share what you are feeling with the care recipient if it seems appropriate and helpful.

*Visit or call or connect online with a close friend or family member to help vent your feelings in a secure and supportive atmosphere.

*Journal about your thoughts and feelings-remember to keep the journal hidden if you are concerned anyone else might read it and take what they read the wrong way.

*Use relaxation strategies to manage stress levels.

*Consult with a professional therapist who can help you understand and deal with your emotions.

*Speak to a chaplain, priest, rabbi, minister, or other religious figure.

*Continue to participate in any spiritual community or practices you might observe.

This leads us to the next area of your life which will be challenged by your transformation into a caregiver. Let's look at the spiritual challenges of caregiving in the next chapter.

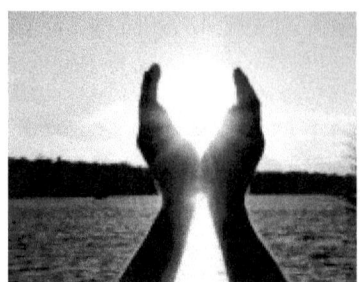

CHAPTER 6
COPING WITH SPIRITUAL CONSIDERATIONS

As a caregiver, you might often question what has happened in your life, and your place in the universe. Meeting your spiritual needs can take a number of forms, and can help you find more emotional balance and inner peace.

Some people enjoy being part of a faith-based community, and attending regular services at a church, temple, or mosque. For others, connections with people can help them feel fulfilled in their role of caregiver, and like they are part of a larger calling.

With certain conditions, however, end of life issues will have to be faced. One's faith can often have an impact on the caregiving process, in particular if their spiritual sense is in conflict with that of the person they are caring for. The issue of death raises a lot of questions about a great unknown for many. Sometimes people who have had faith all their lives suddenly find themselves questioning it. In other cases, people who did not have much spiritual belief find themselves becoming more devout the closer the prospect of death becomes.

Faith is not based on logic, but a complicated web of emotions, beliefs and assumptions. People with faith can often take comfort in it, but having their faith tested and perhaps found lacking in a way they never imagined can lead to many of the negative emotions we discussed in the previous chapter, including anxiety, depression and anger.

Faith can be shaken as soon as a diagnosis is received. "Why me?" is a common question that does not always have a satisfactory answer. In other cases, faith can be renewed or attained, as the care recipient or caregiver gains a sense that they are fulfilling some form of destiny or higher plan.

Faith takes many forms, from a sense of their being a Higher Power, to a general sense of the interconnectedness and sacredness of life. It can be driven by organized religion, attending regular services with a community, or worshiping at home alone through meditation and various rituals.

In order to avoid caregiver burnout, it is important to try to stick to routines that provide comfort and support to you. Prayer, meditation and other acts of devotion can be relaxing and help relieve stress. If your beliefs are at odds with those of your loved one, however, this can cause conflict and stress. It is important to remember that each person has the right to live their own life and also come to terms with their own death in their own way. This might in some cases mean refusing care and treatment, such as giving a Do Not Resuscitate order even if you do not agree with it.

Assisted suicide is a very emotive topic, and in some cases, refusal to continue with medical treatment on the part of the ill person can be seen as suicidal. But it might also be a spiritual belief, based on the thought that the higher power they believe in will either save them, or intends for them to go through the process of illness, or onto whatever afterlife they conceive of.

In other cases, refusal of treatment might also be part of their religious organization, even if it is incomprehensible to us. One of Carolyn's brother's best friends in high school got appendicitis. He was in agony, but his parents refused to take him for medical treatment because they believed in refusing all medical interventions such as surgery or blood transfusions.

Desperate to live, Frank climbed out the window and checked himself into the hospital. He then had the lifesaving surgery, and was in the hospital for a couple of weeks recovering from his close brush with death.

When he was finally able to leave the hospital, and returned home, his parents would not even let him in the door. They told him they were disowning him for defying their beliefs. They had packed his bags, threw them out on the street, and slammed the door in his face. He came to live with Carolyn's family until he graduated and then went to live with an aunt who did not have such extreme beliefs.

Most of us would find these beliefs extreme, and wonder how they could watch their child suffer so much and then never want to have anything to do with them just because they chose to save their own life. Frank was lucky because he was old enough to be allowed to make his own decisions. A younger child would probably have died as a result of the parents' actions.

In other cases, it is the patient themselves that chooses a path of care for themselves based on their faith. Annabelle had a wonderful colleague at her job, Pete, who was funny, intelligent, with a great fiancée and a lovely family. Annabelle and her husband were dating at the time and so the two of them and her friend Pete and his fiancée used to double date.

Things were going great in their lives, but Annabelle noticed that Pete was acting more and more tired. Annabelle also knew her friend did not have the greatest fashion sense, but there seemed to be something odd about the cut of his trousers. One day she said to her husband, "I think Pete is sick." She explained her suspicions, and though it was embarrassing for them all, they managed to get him alone to talk to him about what she thought was going on.

Annabelle had had two other friends become ill and die from testicular cancer. When she and her husband asked Pete if he was suffering from certain symptoms, he admitted he had, but been too embarrassed to go to the doctor. A good Catholic, Pete had never been intimate with his fiancée and knew little about his own body. He noticed the swelling, but assumed it was a sports injury of some sort and would just go away.

The doctor testicular diagnosed cancer and Pete went through the standard surgery, but refused any other treatment, not even taking so much as an aspirin. As time passed, he complained of back pain a great deal, until it got so bad that the doctors finally decided to investigate. Unfortunately, the cancer had spread to the lymph nodes in his back, causing so much pressure that even once they were removed, he had to relearn to walk. Throughout all of this Pete refused any painkillers, determining that the cancer was God's choice for him.

Annabelle and her husband visited Pete every day in the hospital and when he was at home, and were treated like members of the family as they helped with whatever needed to be done. His parents never gave up hope, even though it was clear that Pete was becoming more ill despite all of the doctors' efforts.

One Sunday morning, they were all visiting Pete when the doctor came in with the results of his most recent battery of tests. The doctor told him that the cancer had spread to his liver and brain as well, and that he had about three months left to live.

Pete thanked the doctor, and they all sat discussing next steps for a few moments. The doctor said that if he was willing to finally start using painkillers, they could keep him comfortable until the end. Pete thanked him but refused, saying he was in God's hands and that God would care for him.

After the doctor left, everyone tried to be as positive and upbeat as possible, with his family talking about Pete going to heaven, where he would see his father, who had died the year before after a bout with cancer. Pete was a little bit quiet, and eventually asked them if they could go to the cafeteria for a half an hour so he could just shut his eyes for a few minutes because he had not gotten much sleep the night before.

They all kissed him and went to the cafeteria, where they discussed next steps over a cup of coffee. Then Annabelle heard a Code Blue being called, an emergency, with a patient who needed to be resuscitated. "He's gone, Pete's gone," Annabelle said to her husband.

"What do you mean? We just spoke to him five minutes ago. The doctor said he had three months."

"No, he's gone. He let go. He decided it was time."

Her husband looked at her like she was crazy, but by the time they got back to the room a few moments later, the hospital staff were pronouncing him dead.

His family were naturally sad, but also saw a miracle in his death, him being spared suffering even more months of suffering after all that Pete had endured.

Of course, one could say a lot of the suffering had been self-inflicted. People will often refuse painkillers because they are afraid of becoming addicted, and of course, prescription drug addiction is a risk for people who are not careful.

But the important thing to remember is that even if we are in a position to make care decisions for a loved one, they should not be based solely on our own decisions and religious beliefs, but on theirs. This can cause a great deal of conflict, both outer and inner, but it is a sign of love and respect to do so. If you do not think you can abide by their desires, you should consider allowing someone else to be responsible for carrying out their last wishes.

You should also consider your own arrangements in a similar situation and discuss them with the person you determine to be your next of kin. Through the process of working through these kinds of decisions for yourself, it is possible to gain a lot of valuable insights into the thought processes of your loved one as they work through their own end of life decisions.

Our friend Robert was a very unemotional, matter of fact kind of man until his brother suddenly had a heart attack. Leo had been developmentally challenged all his life, and Robert had become his caregiver a couple of years before, after their father and then mother had died.

Once he had become caregiver, Robert had done everything he could to help Leo become independent and well cared for in case Robert ever died first. But one day Robert got a call saying Leo had had a heart attack. By the time he got to the hospital, they told him that Leo was brain dead, but being kept on life support.

Robert said, "What for, if there is no hope?" and was told that it was up to him to decide whether or not to pull the plug.

Robert also became aware that the hospital staff were keeping Leo on life support because they were hoping to get him to agree to organ donation. Leo was an otherwise healthy man who had been well cared for all his life, and his organs could have made a huge difference to a lot of lives.

But Robert was furious and refused point blank. "The end is the end," he said, "so pull the plug, and allow him to have some peace and dignity in death by not cutting him to pieces. " The very thought of living on a respirator and organ donation horrified him so much, nothing anyone could say could get him to even think through the pros and cons of each situation.

Carolyn's mother has not been to church in years, but still believes in what she was taught as a child, that the body must be complete at the time of death in order to be ready for the Day of Judgment. Her mother will not even consider Carolyn's wanting to donate her organs and be cremated. She persists in this point of view even though the Catholic Church now permits both. Therefore, Carolyn has had to rule her out as someone she would trust to respect her wishes and carry out her final instructions regarding end of life decisions and her final affairs.

Carolyn's father Joe is a Eucharistic minister serving a large Catholic congregation, bringing communion to the elderly, sick, and those who can't get to services regularly, usually because they are suffering from some disability, or caring for someone with health challenges.

Joe attends church every morning and studies his Bible every day. He discusses care and end of life issues with those he visits whenever they ask for his help and for his perspective on their options. He has no qualms at all with Carolyn's end of life decisions. Two parents, two totally different attitudes. But it is all a question of perspective and one's own thoughts about what is 'right' and what isn't.

You can BE right, or you can DO right. It is your decision, of course, but one that your care recipient should also be allowed to make for themselves. If you are caring for someone unable to make those decisions at all, such as a child born with health issues, or someone with a dementing illness, by all means base your decision on your faith if you have one, but balance that with the beliefs of the care recipient, if any, and with the respect and love you would wish to be treated with if you were in the same position.

There are many different perspectives on death, dying and the afterlife. Sometimes exploring these faiths can give a new perspective and even spiritual comfort. Some faiths believe in reincarnation, that we die and are reborn again in this world. For Hindus and Buddhists, karma is the sum of your actions in this life, and these actions will help determine your rebirth in the next. In these faiths, the current body is just a container for the soul, which will move on to a new body once the process of death has been completed in the same way that we would move from one house to another.

Buddhists go for refuge, or seek help from, Buddha, Dharma and Sangha, that is, enlightened beings; the teachings of Buddha, who lived from around 563 BCE to 483 BCE; and spiritual friends.

Buddha is the Sanskrit word for Awakened One, or enlightened one. Buddhism is commonly referred to as the science of the mind, as those who follow the teachings work on perfecting their own mind by following the path to enlightenment. A Buddhist will seek enlightenment in order free themselves and then free others from suffering. In the course of seeking enlightenment, they concentrate on various mental exercises such as meditations, to try to take control of the death and rebirth process. They learn these through the teachings, and seek to live a good life by helping others and sharing their teachings and faith with their spiritual friends.

Through study and meditation, Buddhists try to be conscious at the moment of death in order to be able to remember the lessons from their previous lives. Through remembering all they have learned as they pass from one life to the next, they can gradually get rid of all their bad habits of body, speech and mind, such as eating too much, gossiping, and thinking angry thoughts.

Once they are purified in this way through their working on improving their mind in particular, since it is the controller of all their actions, they will be able to help others through the wisdom they have gained, their new state of enlightenment or Buddhahood. They try to achieve nirvana, not a physical place like Heaven, but a freedom from the endless cycle of birth, death and rebirth.

In order to try to control their rebirth, Buddhists will usually want to be conscious at the moment of their deaths, not loaded with painkillers. They will also want death to take as natural a course as possible, often refusing any treatment at all. This can be difficult for caregivers to understand, especially in a state of the art hospital with so much medical technology available to prolong life.

Again, it is up to the care recipient to determine what is or is not acceptable, based on their own faith or belief system, or not, however much we might be at odds with their choices. We have known Buddhists who have died peacefully without any regrets, and others who have been furiously angry that they wasted their time in this life on unimportant things.

Even if you are not a Buddhist, meditation can be of great benefit in relieving stress and helping you work through challenging issues. Many people think that meditation is all about emptying your mind, but guided Buddhist meditations are usually on one of several topics, such as why we need to work on eliminating the mind of anger, and the nature of existence, birth, aging, sickness and death.

These may not sound like the most cheerful of topics, but many Buddhists and others who have a strong faith will tell you that it is often the moment at which you "know your own death" that you start to travel your spiritual path.

In other words, once a person comes to the realization that they will die one day, they will often try to find ways to make their life meaningful for however short or long a time they are on this Earth. Some might party like rock stars, of course, in an attempt to avoid dealing with the realization, or even commit suicide. Others, however, will usually try to leave something behind. For Buddhists, knowing your time is limited means living mindfully, that is, paying attention to things and looking for practical solutions to everyday problems, so they no longer become problems, but merely challenges to be overcome.

Faith is intensely personal, as are our thoughts on dying, death and possible afterlives, if any. One thing is for sure, though, by connecting with others and allowing them to connect with us, we can feel less alone and fearful of the unknown. Reaching out is one of the best ways to avoid negativity, cope with challenges, and prevent caregiver burn out.

It can also give comfort, such as the stories of people having gone to Heaven, or achieved a good spiritual rebirth, or died peacefully in their sleep.

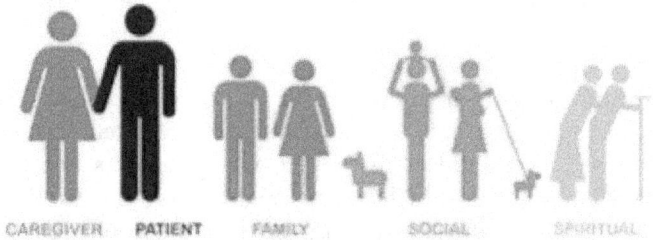

CAREGIVER   PATIENT   FAMILY   SOCIAL   SPIRITUAL

Again, everyone is different, and as a caregiver, you need to try to respect their beliefs even if you do not agree with them. On the other hand, there might be some comfort in the thought that the end of one thing really is just the beginning of another, with even better things to look forward to in the future. That death is a part of life, and that if we think about it, our loved one will always be with us through our memories of them, even if they are no longer present physically.

Think about it: Even if your father dies, he does not stop being your father, does he? The time shared, lessons taught and learned, are all still with you to the end of your life.

In most cases, our caregiving will be temporary and of a limited duration, with a good prognosis. We hope this is the case for you on your caregiver journey. But even if of only short duration and a happy outcome, caregiving can still be the most emotionally and spiritually challenging situation you will ever face, with few answers to your many questions.

The important thing to remember is that no matter what you do or do not believe, you need to manage your stress levels and those of your care recipient. You also need to balance your cares and concerns with those of your loved one, and respect their point of view and wishes even if you do not agree with them or even understand them.

Faith and belief, or lack thereof, are not things that can easily be explained or changed through discussion, but they can bring comfort to the sick and to caregivers. Do whatever you feel most comfortable with in respect to your own faith. It might also help to remember that in almost every major religion, love for others is considered to be an important value, if not the highest one, from Christian to Buddhist to Hindu and more.

Many people think love is just an emotion, but it is an active choice we make each day with all the people around us, showing that we care in a range of ways in order to preserve harmonious relationships. From our colleagues at work to our loved ones at home, the little actions we do can all add up to the message that they are important in our lives and that we value them.

In the stressful situation of caregiving, we can sometimes lose sight of the little things. And in the stress of caregiving, we are often confronted with some really big questions that even the greatest scholars and philosophers in the world do not have any answers for. Because in fact, each of us needs to find our own answer, by listening to our inner truth.

Support your loved one in your caregiving role as much as you can, but be sure to get the emotional and spiritual support you need too on your caregiving journey. Also be prepared to demand the same support and respect yourself if you are ever in a position of needing to be cared for one day. Ask for help as and when you need it in order to avoid caregiver burnout, no matter where that help comes from. Accept the help you receive with gratitude, even if it does not take the form you might imagine.

One of the more stressful aspects of caregiving after a loved one has had an accident or becomes ill is having to deal with the whole host of strangers you suddenly find in your life, namely doctors, nurses and other health care workers. How you deal with them directly influences how they deal with you, and can be a cause of further stress, or helpful support. Let's look in the next chapter at dealing with health care workers.

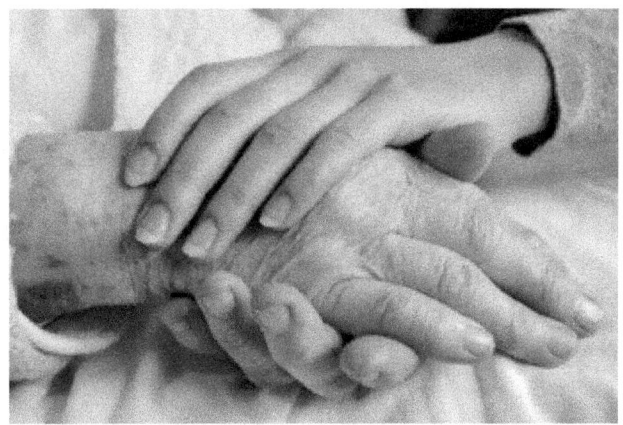

CHAPTER 7
COPING WITH DOCTORS, HOSPITAL STAFF AND OTHER HEALTHCARE WORKERS

In the United States, we are rapidly approaching a health care crisis, with an aging population, stressed out health care workers, and a system stretched to breaking point in terms of resources available, and demand on resources.

Most of us have an image of hospitals being clean, restful places where an injured or sick person will be cared for well in the hope of a good outcome. Unfortunately, this is becoming a rarity, rather than a norm.

Doctors have more patients to see than ever and really can't go over their allocated 15 minutes if they want to make enough money in their practice and not back up their schedule for hours at a time. One of our local GPs regularly keeps patients waiting an average of 2 to 3 hours even early in the morning because he schedules so many and gets so backed up. His staff are so disorganized that even when lab results come in, they are not acted upon. The patient gets no follow up call, and they are lucky if the right lab results actually get filed in the correct folder. We have reported him time and again for doing a disservice to the community, but so far nothing has been done to get him to clean up his act.

Then we have the hospital emergency room, with burned out nurses rushed off their feet and so lacking in compassion that they leave patients laying in their own diarrhea for 8 hours at a time. Our friend got an E. coli infection as a result of this neglect and nearly died because they also neglected to give her the antibiotics that she had been prescribed.

Those who do try to run a tight ship do so at their own cost, suffering from burnout and 'compassion fatigue', just getting the job done, but with little to no 'human touch' in their caregiving. They go through the motions like robots, and stick to protocol to the letter without ever taking the trouble to explain what is going on to a sick or scared patient or caregiver.

If your loved one ends up in a long-term care situation, you might have a health worker come to you home to assist you. Our friend Grace got one after her husband had a stroke. The woman ate almost everything that was in the refrigerator, seemed to always be 'on break' whenever Grace asked her to do anything, and helped herself to the contents of Grace's jewelry box on her way out. No one ever saw her again and the police were never able to recover the stolen items.

Hospitals and nursing homes are full of germs, which are spread from patient to patient by careless workers who do not wash their hands or use gloves, or who rely on hand sanitizer even though it only kills about 97% of known germs. Hospital infections are on the rise, with many of them life-threatening. Frank McCourt, the author of Angela's Ashes, died of meningitis that he acquired in a hospice setting. Viral pneumonia is a common cause of death in elderly patients who have been bed-ridden for some time, such as after hip replacement surgery.

Our friend Mike's son Chris caught MRSA, Methacillin-Resistant Staphylococcus Aureus, the 'flesh-eating bug', as a newborn, and had to be bathed at least twice a day and rinsed down with a special solution to try to stop the MRSA from penetrating into his skin and attacking.

All of these horror stories are not the norm, it is true, but we are offering them as a reminder that just because people are working in the medical profession does not make them infallible, and does not mean that they have your loved one's best interests at heart.

From our own experience, we have seen that those patients who have regular visitors who stay around at the hospital and take an active interest in what is going on are much less likely to be neglected than, for example, a frail, elderly person with few or no family members who does not dare ask questions or complain if there is a problem.

If your loved one is able to speak up for themselves, great, but if they are not, this job will fall to you as the primary caregiver, and this chore can be very stressful and lead to burnout if you are not careful.

Again, we are not talking about perfectionism here, or asking staff to go above and beyond the call of duty. But at the very least, we should expect them to their jobs in a prompt, courteous and professional manner, with the well-being of the patient, not themselves, in mind.

Whenever we have encountered staff with a bad attitude, we have not confronted them directly. Instead, we have said, "Thank you for everything you are doing. I can see that you take your job seriously and care for your patients the same way you would want your Mother (Father/Sister/Brother etc) to be cared for."

Most of the time, it works, and you see an improvement in the care. Only the workers with real caregiver burnout or those who see it as 'just a job' will not correct themselves.

Because yes, even professionals get caregiver burnout and suffer from 'compassion fatigue', in which they mentally and even physically distance themselves from the patients they are meant to be caring for, retreating to their computers, paperwork and so on and never even bringing a bedpan, or leaving them sitting on it for hours, while they look at their watch and calculate the number of hours until their shift is over.

It is a sad state of affairs, but one driven by the need to keep costs down even as more and more people get ill. For example, 2015 is shaping up to be one of the worst cold and flu seasons ever due to the vaccination not covering the dominant strains that have been spreading. Carolyn was in the ER with family twice in the past 2 weeks, and it was like a vision of hell, with every bed taken and stretcher too. Those who should have been moved up to rooms were not able to do so because there were none, and then they began to start using every wheel chair in order to free up the stretchers so the ambulances could unload still more critically ill patients being brought in.

Admittedly this is New York City, so the demand is high for health services, but that demand has been driven still higher by several hospitals having closed, such as St. Vincent's, which was run into the ground by its own foolish managers. Any hospital closure creates a domino effect, and more patients and stress on the system mean more stress on the health care workers.

So what can you as a caregiver do when confronted with overworked, underpaid and stressed out healthcare workers? Be reasonable, but firm. Ask for what you need, and if they are not willing or able to give it, see what you can do to secure it for yourself. That may be information, a pillow, fresh sheets or pee pads for the bed, whatever.

Keep receipts for EVERYTHING you buy or spend that are related to caregiving, including receipts for car service, gas back and forth, supplies and so on. Once a person has spent more than 10% of their income on health-related costs, such as co-pays travel, and so on, the expenses can be itemized and deducted from your taxes.

Keep records of what happened. If you are having trouble with a particular member of staff, find out their name and later, when the crisis is over, write a letter of complaint stating exactly what happened. Stick to the facts without being insulting or accusatory. Many hospitals now have 'risk management specialists who take these complaints seriously if only to avoid being sued by patients and family members who are not receiving an appropriate standard of care.

If a health agency sends a home health worker or other member of staff to assist you in your home, check them out fully, and ask the agency how closely they investigate their workers to make sure they are the real deal and not some con woman like Grace ended up with. In these days of the Internet, it is easy to look up information on almost anyone, so there is no excuse for agencies not bothering and just hiring 'a warm body' when in fact health care workers are supposed to possess nursing skills and honesty and integrity.

Any new person coming to our home can be intrusive, but particularly when you are already stressed over a health situation. Set boundaries that are clear, such as when their breaks are, and who is providing their lunch, dinner, and so on. They should provide all they need for themselves.

Coffee, tea and water can be provided within reason, but they should not be helping themselves any time they feel like it. They are there to work and offer care, not put their feet up and watch you while you run yourself ragged. If there are any issues you are not happy about, speak to them directly regarding the nature of the complaint and what solutions you would suggest. If things do not improve, call the agency to discuss the matter. Again, keep records of what was done, said and so on. The person with the best records is the person who will win their case in most instances, and get the outcome they wish for.

In most cases, we have been fortunate enough to end up with helpers who have become friends, and even like members of the family. Ask around your circle of family and friends in your area to see if there is anyone that they would recommend as a nurse, companion, childminder, and so on. Also ask about cleaning help and any other services that can make your life easier so you are not trying to do everything yourself, which is a recipe for burnout.

Consider a range of options when caring for your loved one. For example, if you know a stay at home mom next door to you, see if she might be willing to look in on him, check to see he is eating 3 meals a day, or if she would be willing to have him in her own home while you are at work so he is not all alone for 10 hours a day. See if there is elder day care in your area, or if physical therapist can come to the house regularly instead of you needing to drive them everywhere for appointments.

In some cases, retired nurses are available for home health work. Others might work on their days off, or volunteer to help families in need to ensure their loved ones got round the clock care. When our neighbor Mitch was very ill, he got two very nice healthcare workers who were only being paid for 8 hours by the agency, but were willing to work an extra 4 hours off the books for a very reasonable sum in order to ensure that he was never on his own.

Maybe someone in your family works in the health industry, or knows someone who does. Assess your needs depending on the accident, illness or prognosis, and fill in any gaps in the care plan with one or more helpers or volunteers who can pick up the slack.

Be clear about what you need, what is available, and what you can afford to supplement any services, and again, do not try to do it all yourself. You are the quarterback. You do not need to personally score every touchdown.

We hope you will not have your already stressful situation added to by an outside health worker with attitude, but if you do encounter this, nip it in the bud before it ever gets out of hand so you are not the one who ends up suffering as you get more stressed and burned out.

Sometimes despite everything we do, we are forced to start considering and discussing end of life decisions. to make end of life in relation to our loved one. Let's look at this topic in the next chapter.

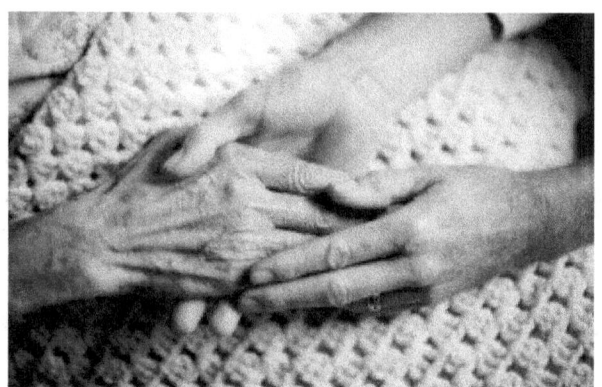

CHAPTER 8
COPING WITH END OF LIFE DECISIONS

Of course we all hope that our loved one will recover after an accident or illness, but in some cases, despite everyone's best efforts, end of life decisions will have to be faced. This is of course only natural for all of us, for none of us can live forever, but most people want to avoid thinking about the topic of their own death for as long as possible, and in many cases, leave it until it is too late.

Some people say it is morbid to think about it, while others realize that where there is life, there will be death sooner or later. The main consideration here should be respecting the wishes of the loved one as far as possible, and trying to avoid leaving behind a lot of chaos and confusion for those who remain behind.

There are a lot of emotional aspects to death, of course, but also legal and financial ones as well that need to be taken care of sooner rather than later in some cases. One of our friends recently went through a diagnosis of cancer with her mother. From the time they discovered it, gave her treatment, and she died, was a matter of weeks. Every time they tried to discuss end of life issues, her father would say, "We're not THERE yet." But suddenly, they WERE, and no one was prepared.

In the Unites States, every state has different laws with respect to wills, living wills, end of life decisions, and what happens if someone is ill or dies without any legal paperwork with reference to their wishes having been created and organized in such a way as to be legally binding.

When bad things happen to us, we may feel at the time as if we are the only person in the world who is going through these things. The truth is that many people have been caregivers before and experienced end of life issues, and so there are professionals and other supportive people at hand who are there to help if and when you need it.

The idea of organizing a funeral, for example, can seem overwhelming, but many establishments package together cost-effectively the essentials that most families require, leaving you with only a few decisions to be made, such as the casket, urn, and so forth. Take all the good advice you can and draft in as much help as possible at each stage of the process.

None of us want to think about death and dying, but the truth is a will and living will, if filed correctly, can make things a great deal easier for all concerned, especially the caregiver, and any other people affected by the illness and eventual death of the loved one. Assigning one person to serve as the 'proxy' (prock-SEE) to make important care decisions can mean more timely decision making and intervention if needed. Read through the useful booklet at http://www.caringinfo.org/files/public/brochures/End-of-Life_Decisions.pdf with your loved one in order to be clear about these issues and put arrangements into place for BOTH of you. Being prepared makes things a great deal easier for everyone concerned.

It can also mean that if the patient states that they wish a Do Not Resuscitate (DNR) order if their heart stops, for example, that this wish will also be respected. There are a range of examples online of wills and living wills which you and your loved one can use as the models for your own. Be sure to have them signed and witnessed by independent parties who would not benefit from the wills in any way, and do try to have them put on file correctly depending on the state you are in.

Dying intestate (in-TEST-ate), that is, without a legally binding will, can make things very difficult and stressful for the person having to make plans and arrangements for a funeral, for example, and for what is termed estate management, that is, dealing with the property of the deceased. Illness and death are already stressful enough without also having to worry about money and legal entanglements, so if your loved one has not already made their wishes known, it will be important to get ready to have a conversation about this subject.

>In terms of funeral arrangements and so on, as we have already

discussed, some people favor burials, others cremation. With the average funeral costing $17,000 these days, be sure you are aware of their wishes, the estimated costs, and any special requirements both for your state, and for the cemetery, for example, where you loved one will be laid to rest.

For instance, if your loved one was a veteran, they would be entitled to certain considerations, but the cemetery might have more strict rules and regulations as a result. Carolyn's uncle at Pinelawn National Cemetery, for example, received an honor guard when he died, but the cemetery only allows bronze plaques, not head stones, and only cut flowers in the vase that is part of the plaque, not plants of any kind. Knowing the rules up front can help avoid distress, stress and wasted money and effort.

It is only natural to want to do the best for your loved one and respect their wishes, but don't aim for an impossible standard of perfection and then feel as though you have let anyone done. Keep to the spirit of what they would have wanted, and what you can realistically afford if you have to pay for it yourself, or what insurance will cover. Also keep in mind that you will usually have to pay the expenses up front and then get reimbursed, so plan accordingly.

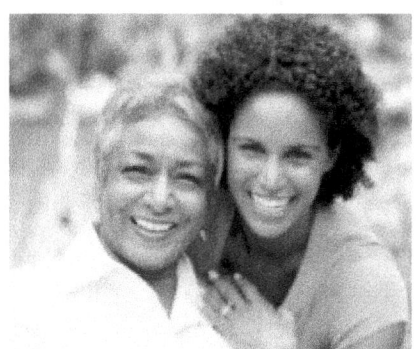

CONCLUSION

Coping with a loved one's physical or mental challenges is difficult for anyone to have to face. An accident or illness will usually occurs quite suddenly, leaving you wondering what hit you.

The shock of having a child with a disability, a parent starting to decline in their faculties, or a loved one being in an accident or getting diagnosed with a serious illness can be some of the hardest things anyone has to face in life.

Our first reaction is that we don't want our loved one to go through their life without support from someone who cares for them. However, it can also be a decision made with emotions and not enough facts, leading people to fear the worst or throw them into the role of primary caregiver without any idea of what will be required, how long it will last, or how they can care for themselves to avoid caregiver burnout.

Helping a loved one can be very difficult at first because they have to adjust as well. This can also lead to a lot of stress and tension in the household. Money worries, plus emotional considerations such as anxiety, depression, anger, guilt and grief at the loss of your old life can also come into play in both of your lives.

When faced with any caregiving situation, the first thing to do is to learn all you can about the diagnosis and the prognosis for your loved one. In this way you will know where you are going, and can start to develop a plan in conjunction with all the medical personnel who might be involved with your loved one's medical condition. This plan will help you and other family members adequately plan for a loved one's care now and in the future, however long or short that future may be. It can also help you feel in more control of what happening and make your ride on the emotional rollercoaster of caregiving a smoother one with fewer deep downward plunges.

You will probably want to spend a lot of time with your loved one out of concern that they will need you, but pace yourself. If this is to be a long-term condition, do what you can to foster independence as far as is reasonable. There is no need to sacrifice your entire life to help your loved one. You can be there for them in terms of time, support, financial aid, moral support, or all of the foregoing, but you don't always have to be right in the same room with them.

Try to maintain the friendships and the activities that you enjoyed before you started to be a caregiver, so you can continue to lead your own life even as you help your loved one.

Above all, don't neglect your health because you are caring for another. If they are relying on you, you want to be the best you can be, not a burned out wreck, or worse still, sick yourself with some illness or chronic medical condition. Be sure to go for an annual check-up, regular trips to the dentist, well woman clinics and so on. An ounce of prevention is worth a pound of cure, in most cases.

Eating right, exercising and being sure to get enough rest are the best ways to avoid caregiver burnout and be in top shape to help your loved one and still lead your own satisfying life. Use this guide to help remind yourself of the warning signs of caregiving, and practical action steps you can take to care for yourself and your loved one. We have summarized the essential action steps below for your convenience. Also make sure you use the chapter on emotions to give yourself a 'checkup from the neck up' so any negative emotion you might be feeling do not get out of control. Use the list of signs and symptoms to spot any trouble areas, and the strategies to help deal with the negative emotion.

Here's wishing you, your loved one and your family the best as you cope with your caregiving.
C.S.
A.S.
December 3, 2016

FURTHER READING

All Eternal Spiral Books titles are available to buy, and to read through the Kindle Unlimited Program-millions of books, one low monthly fee.

We offer a range of healthy living guides through the Health Matters series. http://eternalspiralbooks.com/category/categories-series/health

All our titles are available through Kindle Unlimited as well. Millions of books available for one low monthly fee.

We also offer a range of free ecourses you can sign up for to help you with a range of health and wellness topics.
http://eternalspiralbooks.com/list/

ACTION STEPS CHECKLIST

Here's a checklist of action steps based on what you have learned in each chapter.

When dealing with any caregiving issue, you will need to know:

*The diagnosis

*The prognosis (possible outcome)

*What care will be required, when and for how long

*How to deal with the loved one after the diagnosis, both physically and mentally

*How to deal with your own self-care issues

*How to plan for the future given the prognosis.

CHAPTER 1: DEALING WITH THE CRISIS AND DIAGNOSIS

* Learn all you can about the illness or condition in order to work as a team with your loved one and his/her medical team.

* Learn how to deal with the new normal in your life.

* Learn to give up on ideas of perfect and accept good enough.

CHAPTER 2: DEVELOPING A CARE PLAN

* Research various places that you and your loved one might be able to get more help, including:

- Churches

- Charitable foundations (Make a Wish, Ronald McDonald House, etc.)

- Organizations and charities dedicated to that illness

- Hospitals

- The Federal government

- Pharmaceutical companies and their charitable divisions

- Medical schools and their researchers

- Hospitals

* Assemble your team and support network from among family members and friends.

* Learn to delegate.

* Learn to ask for help when you need it.

* Connect with other caregivers online or in person.

* Use your local hospital as a resource for information and support, as needed.

* Be sure you understand all instructions given upon your loved one leaving the hospital.

* Don't be shy about asking questions.

* Don't think you are taking up too much of their valuable time with reference to medical staff.

* Determine your loved one's situation with regard to short-term and long-term care insurance.

* Determine your loved one's situation with regard to disability insurance.

* Determine your loved one's situation with regard to Social Security.

* Be sure to stay on top of your finances and those of your loved one at this time.

* Stay in touch with the health insurance company to make sure they give pre-approval for treatment and know what is going on.

* Stay in touch with your auto insurance company if the loved one was injured as a result of an accident.

* Try to deal with your loved one's care on a whole family basis, with everyone doing their share.

* Try to give your loved one age-appropriate care, for example, if they are a senior or a child.

CHAPTER 3: DEALING WITH A LOVED ONE INDIVIDUALLY

* If your loved one is in the hospital, prepare as much as possible for their homecoming.

* Ask the professionals about adaptive devices and equipment, if needed, to get your home ready.

* If you are only renting your home, consider moving to a place that will be better suited to the needs of the person requiring care.

* If you need to care for an elderly parent, discuss the most practical living arrangements that can be found from among everyone in the family. Then make sure the others get involved, each in their own way, to help.

* If the illness or injury is temporary, remind yourself of this.

* If the illness or injury is permanent, try to negotiate a new normal with your family.

* Deal with denial in your loved one and yourself quickly; facing facts can lead to a better outcome.

* Watch out for signs of depression.

* Allow yourself to grieve for the things you and your loved one have lost, but also realize that your new life will be good, just different.

* If your loved one's prognosis is not good, deal with end-of-life issues as best you can.

* Don't be afraid to ask for professional help with respect to end-of-life issues and your feelings about them.

* Try to affect positive changes that will help the whole family stay as healthy as possible.

* Keep everyone informed so that they can be vigilant and also help as needed.

* Understand that sometimes your loved one's moods are the result of the illness, not anything you have done.

* Understand that sometimes your love one might become frustrated and take it out on you because you are the nearest person they can do so with.

* Understand that your loved one will test your limits, consciously or unconsciously, to see how much you care.

* Deal with any very bad behavior by either ignoring it and going about your business, or telling the person that it is unacceptable.

* Try to maintain your boundaries and respect those of your loved one even if you are acting as their caregiver.

* Learn as much as you can about the condition, and what is typical for sufferers, so you can also learn how to deal with these issues.

* Give tough love as needed.

* Avoid feeling guilty. None of this is your fault.

* With children who need caregiving, still try to discipline them in the same manner as you would any other child.

* Try to make every member of the family participate as much as possible according to their own abilities.

* Value each contribution and effort.

* In terms of caregiving, understand that people have different capacities in terms of time, skills, and money.

* Learn to leverage people's times, skills and/or money as part of a long-term care plan for the loved one.

* Welcome all help, no matter how great or small.

* Encourage the loved one to maintain a healthy circle of friends and participate in various activities.

* You should also maintain a healthy circle of friends and participate in a variety of activities.

* If you are part of a couple, make sure you have regular date nights and breaks from caregiving, to help you relax and re-charge your batteries.

CHAPTER 4: TAKING CARE OF THE CAREGIVER

* Be sure not to neglect your own health while looking after a loved one.

* Learn to delegate.

* Get help with regular household chores that anyone can do.

* Get rid of the "do it yourself is best" mentality.

* Exercise every day.

* Try to go for a walk outside each day for some fresh air.

* If it is hard to get outside due to the nature of your loved one's condition, set up a small home gym/workout area and rent some workout DVDs.

* Eat nutritious food.

* Try to get high-quality sleep every night.

* Do something every day that you enjoy.

* Make time to de-stress and relax.

* Take a multivitamin if you think you need one.

* Beware of cold and flu. If your loved one is dependent on you, consider getting a flu shot each season.

* Join a support group to help get emotional support.

* Avoid caregiver burnout.

* Use the Internet as a valuable tool for information, support and advice.

CHAPTER 5: DEALING WITH EMOTIONS

*Caregiving can be very rewarding provided you stay balanced

*Enjoy your positive emotions

*Recognize negative emotions but don't dwell on them

*Consider journaling about your feelings

*Understand that caregiving will naturally result in feelings of
worry
guilt
grief
and so on, but you don't need to let these feelings overwhelm you.

*Learn positive coping strategies

*Avoid negative coping strategies like alcohol and tobacco

*Learn how to manage your stress

*Learn when to speak up and when it is best to remain silent

*Don't worry about 'should' and 'shouldn't'

CHAPTER 6: DEALING WITH SPIRITUAL CONSIDERATIONS

*Death is a important topic in all religions

*So too mght be medical care, such as transfusions, stem cells and so on

*Discuss your thought and feeling with your loved one

*Listen as they discuss theirs

*Consider trying meditation, such as mindfulness meditation. Learn more
with the help of this video:
http://eternalspiralbooks.com/mindfulness-course-101-video/

CHAPTER 7: DEALING WITH HOSPITAL STAFF AND OTHER
HELPERS

*Keep a notebook of questions, things to do and so on

*Don't be afraid to get a second opinion

*Do your own research

*Connect with others online and offline to come up with a care plan that really works for your loved one, and for you

CHAPTER 8: DEALING WITH END OF LIFE DECISIONS

*Deal with practical end of life issues sooner rather than later

*There are many forms to fill out that can make the entire process a lot easier

*Discuss your options with a hospitalist or other professional

*Be sure you are clear about what arrangements each person in your family, including yourself, would like to have, based on their religious beliefs and personal preferences

*No one ever like to think about death, but it is hard to handle these practical matters when you are completely overcome by grief